Aesthetic and Functional Labiaplasty

Stefan Gress

Aesthetic and Functional Labiaplasty

Springer

Stefan Gress
Plastic and Reconstructive Surgery
Munich
Germany
Lucian-Blaga University Sibiu (ULBS) Romania

ISBN 978-3-319-86810-3 ISBN 978-3-319-60222-6 (eBook)
DOI 10.1007/978-3-319-60222-6

Softcover re-print of the Hardcover 1st edition 2017

Printed on acid-free paper

This Springer imprint is published by Springer Nature
The registered company is Springer International Publishing AG
The registered company address is: Gewerbestrasse 11, 6330 Cham, Switzerland

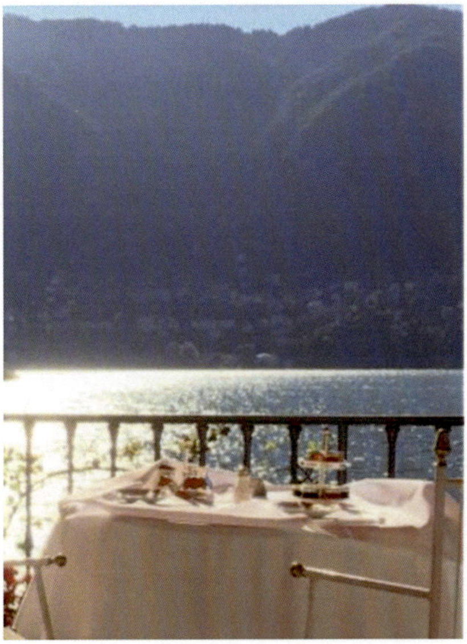

For my happiest time I shared with Janette

Foreword

It may seem a little strange that I, a gynaecologist, am writing a foreword to commend a book by a plastic surgeon. But I feel the need to comment on this key contribution from someone with such in-depth knowledge of the anatomy of the female external genitalia and the surgery of associated deformities.

Not infrequently, unusually large labia minora are bothersome in today's popular sporting activities such as cycling, horse riding, ballet, and other activities where women wear tight-fitting workout clothes and sports gear.

As intimate shaving has become an integral part of personal hygiene, more focus is being placed on the vulva as a feature of a woman's external appearance. For this reason, women who are not happy with this aspect of their appearance often avoid visiting public saunas, for example.

The changes in sexual behaviour in our time—when the sexual experience itself is more important than aspects of reproduction—mean that the vulva is now perceived as part of the body image much more than even a few years ago. Some women obviously find that enlarged labia minora do not fit their ideal body image and sometimes regard them as physical deformities.

In routine practice, gynaecologists are increasingly being confronted with this problem, which affects quite a large number of women. With a lack of standardised surgical procedures to treat functional and aesthetic aspects of vulval anatomy, however, affected women find that their complaints are trivialised, not taken seriously, or, in the worst case, ignored completely.

Vulval anatomy shows great variability, both congenital and acquired from injuries sustained during childbirth. In particular, asymmetrical or greatly enlarged labia minora can distort the body image so permanently that the woman's sex life can be seriously affected. Doctors who empathise with their patients will surely understand their desire for correction.

Professor Gress has studied the anatomy of the female external genitalia in great depth. This book is the result of his intensive involvement with possible surgical corrections, taking both aesthetic and functional aspects into consideration. A surgical technique that spares the erogenous zones of the vulva is essential for a good aesthetic and functional outcome. His excellent results are so far removed from the "labiaplasties" which are unfortunately all too often substandard and which should better be left untreated. In the interests of all those women who are affected and are indeed suffering, I hope therefore that this welcome monograph will be widely distributed amongst plastic surgeons and concerned gynaecologists.

Munich, Germany
November 2016

Werner Albrich

Preface

Under the heading of "Intimate Surgery", procedures to reshape the female external genitalia and improve both appearance and function have greatly increased in popularity in the Western world.

My specialist training as a plastic surgeon started in 1994 in the Department of Plastic and Reconstructive Surgery at the *Klinikum rechts der Isar* university hospital in Munich, under the aegis of Prof. Biemer and Dr. Schaff. During that time, the surgical team was performing complex genital procedures on both men and women in routine practice, especially sex reassignment surgery in transsexualism.

On one occasion, a woman suffering from very long and, in her own words, "repulsive" inner vaginal lips presented to our outpatient clinic. She told us that she had never let her husband see her naked in all their years of marriage, which had put a considerable strain on their sex life and their relationship. At that time, we performed a wedge resection using the technique published by Dr. Gary Alter, working in Los Angeles.

After more and more women came to consult me following another case reported on television later on, by which time I had set up my own practice in Munich, I began to think about this technique with respect to my patients' expectations on the aesthetic results. In particular, these women wanted their inner labia to be completely covered by the outer labia. But this simply wasn't possible with the wedge resection method. So I developed my own technique, which differed from the previously published methods in that not only did it reduce the labia minora below the clitoris but it also reshaped labial tissue in the region of the clitoral hood and the part above. In addition, any protrusion of the clitoris could be corrected.

Over the years, I have modified and refined this technique, to meet the growing aesthetic demands of the ever-increasing number of women requesting surgery.

At the start of my career in female genital cosmetic surgery, almost all of the requests were for labia minora reductions, but, possibly due to media coverage of the emerging medical possibilities, the range of requests has since widened to cover the whole spectrum of intimate surgery.

Other procedures include remodelling the labia majora by tightening up lax skin or by volume augmentation, sculpturing the mons pubis, hymen reconstruction surgery, and operations to restore or improve the response to sexual stimulation, e.g. G-spot amplification, vaginal reshaping, and tightening of the pelvic floor, especially after childbirth.

This book, however, is intended to address only improvements in the shape and function of the external genitalia.

I have placed the greatest emphasis on techniques for reducing the labia minora, as these operations account for well over 60% of all intimate surgery.

As the number of aesthetically unacceptable results due to inadequate surgery is unfortunately also on the increase, especially with reduction labiaplasties, I have included a chapter dedicated to the possibilities of labia minora reconstruction. Reconstruction of such iatrogenic deformities has meanwhile become a sorry routine in my practice. One reason for these botched operations may be the current lack of surgical standards for intimate surgery in the textbooks on plastic surgery and gynaecology. Another reason may be an underestimation of the procedures involved in female genital cosmetic surgery. Labia minora reductions, in particular, are often viewed as trivial procedures with the approach "we'll soon snip that off".

Even more than any other area of the female anatomy, the genital area deserves special attention. It is not only a matter of improving shape and function by overcoming bothersome or disturbing factors, but it is also a question of maintaining or even increasing sensitivity for moments and situations that are some of the highlights of our human existence and for which we are usually prepared to make every possible effort.

If we, as doctors and surgeons, want to devote ourselves to this field, we should set to work with nothing less than this full appreciation of the issues concerned.

With my experience and reflections, I hope that I can make a small contribution to future successes and would be delighted to think that this book will be a helpful companion for my colleagues.

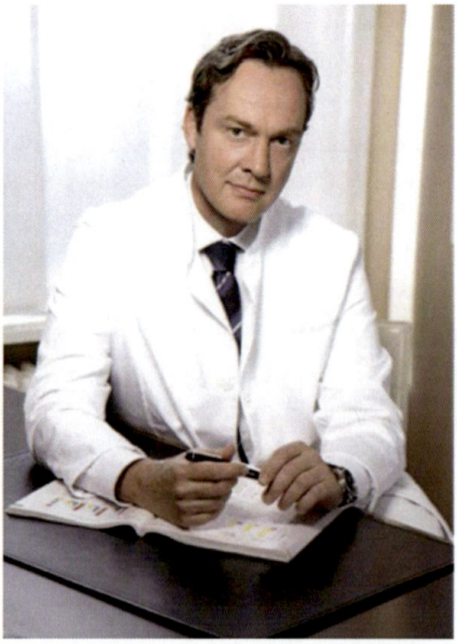

Munich, Germany Stefan Gress

Acknowledgements

Being invited to write this book was a great honour for me. First and foremost, therefore, my thanks go to the publishers, Axel Springer Publisher, Springer International, and in particular to Dr. Inga von Behrens for her confidence in me.

No pathway to success is possible without the support of those nearest and dearest. A big thank you to my parents, Werner and Christa, who have always encouraged and supported me in my professional career, and to my children, Antonia, Lenny, and David, whose time I stole to write this book. I see them little enough as it is, so I am grateful for their patience and understanding.

Special thanks go to my colleague, Prof. Werner Albrich, with whom I have been working for many years and for whom I have the greatest esteem on both a personal and professional level. My whole practice team deserves my gratitude and praise for their support and endless patience with a boss who was occasionally somewhat under stress.

I am particularly indebted to Prof. Di Marino in Marseilles, France, for his help with questions of anatomy. His book *Anatomic Study of the Clitoris and the Bulbo-Clitoral Organ* has been a substantial guideline for my work.

I would also like to register my appreciation of the teachers and trainers during my specialist training, especially Prof. Biemer, whom I have to thank for my inclusion in the world of plastic surgery, and Dr. Jürgen Schaff, who was my esteemed and patient mentor.

My thanks also go to Prof. Glenn Jelks and Prof. Sherrell Aston in New York, as well as to the late Prof. Ivo Pitanguy in Rio de Janeiro, all of whom inspired me with the awesome perfection which they made look deceptively easy and who have been role models for me ever since I started working in this wonderful profession.

Words cannot express my gratitude to Prof. Adriana Stanila and Prof. Rodica Miclea and the Medical Faculty of Sibiu University (ULBS) in Romania for their continuing support.

And last, but not least, writing this book would not have been possible without the confidence of all my patients coming to my clinic for surgery. Thank you to all of them.

Contents

Practical Surgical Anatomy

In any surgical procedure, precise knowledge of the relevant anatomy is of key importance for a successful outcome.

A guiding principle of surgery in the genital area is to maintain sensation under all circumstances. Everything else is secondary to this main maxim. What is the use of an aesthetically pleasing result if the ability to respond to sexual stimulation has been reduced even marginally? In refreshing your memory of the anatomy, therefore, I have paid particular attention to demonstrating and describing the nerve supply, especially that of the clitoris.

Pelvic Floor

The pelvic floor consists of sheets of muscle and connective tissue. Its main function is to hold the abdominal and pelvic organs in place. Openings in the centre allow the intestine, vagina, and urethra to pass through.

The main part of the pelvic floor, the pelvic diaphragm, is formed largely by the levator ani muscle. The smaller part that extends between the ischial rami and the inferior pubic rami is called the urogenital diaphragm: it is formed by the trapezoidal deep transverse perineal muscle.

The openings where the vagina and urethra pass through the urogenital diaphragm are surrounded by the ring of the urethrovaginal sphincter muscle. This sheet of muscle lies between the inferior fascia of the urogenital diaphragm (the perineal membrane) on its lower surface and the superior fascia of the urogenital diaphragm on its upper surface. These two fasciae unite at the apex of the muscle layer to form the transverse perineal ligament (Krause ligament), forming the anterior part of the urogenital diaphragm. Here there is a small cleft between the urogenital diaphragm and the inferior pubic ligament (arcuate ligament) as it arches across the subpubic angle, through which the deep dorsal clitoral vein passes to drain into the vesical venous plexus (*bulbs*). The vein is accompanied by the cavernous nerves, which unite with the dorsal clitoral nerves after leaving the cleft.

S. Gress, *Aesthetic and Functional Labiaplasty*,
DOI 10.1007/978-3-319-60222-6_1

The inferior aspect of the perineal membrane is covered by a layer of connective tissue, the superficial perineal fascia (Colles' fascia). The superficial perineal region lies in between.

Running transversely from the ischial tuberosity to the central tendon of the perineum (perineal body) are the fibres of the superficial transverse perineal muscle, a superficial muscle that is only poorly developed in women.

(The posterior part of the urogenital diaphragm is formed by the trapezoidal deep transverse perineal muscle.)

The connective tissue of the central tendon of the perineum (perineal body) is located at the transition between the urogenital diaphragm and the pelvic diaphragm in the middle of the pelvic floor; it lies between the anus and the posterior commissure. The central tendon of the perineum is a mass of interlocking muscular, fascial, and fibrous components, including the tendons of the levator ani and the deep and superficial transverse perineal muscles. Mechanically speaking, the perineal body is an important junction of the pelvic floor (Fig. 1).

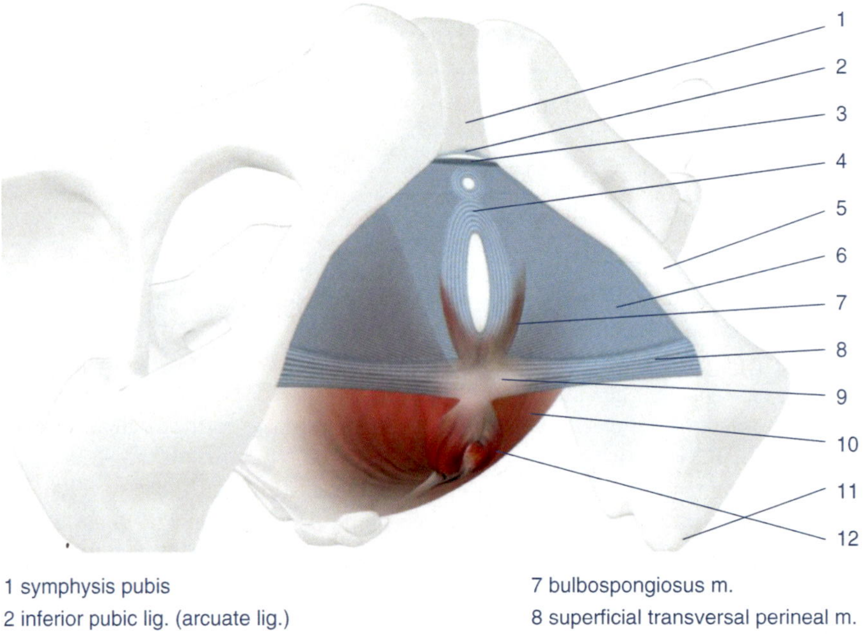

1 symphysis pubis
2 inferior pubic lig. (arcuate lig.)
3 transverse perineal lig. (*Krause* lig.)
4 urethrovaginal m.
5 inferior ischio-pubic ramus
6 deep transversal perineal m. (urogenital diaphragm)
7 bulbospongiosus m.
8 superficial transversal perineal m.
9 tendinous center of the perineum (perineal body)
10 levator ani m.
11 ischial tuberosity
12 external anal sphincter m.

Fig. 1 Urogenital diaphragm

Vulva

The vulva (pudendum) includes all of the following structures: labia majora, labia minora, clitoris, vaginal vestibule, urinary meatus, corpora spongiosa (vestibular bulbs), and the mons pubis (Fig. 2).

Labia Majora

The labia majora (outer labia, large outer vaginal lips) are a pair of prominent folds of the skin that lie together in a gentle curve around the labia minora. They extend from the mons pubis to the perineum. They are joined anteriorly and posteriorly by bridges of tissue—the anterior and posterior commissures. Anteriorly the labia majora merge almost seamlessly into the mons pubis and posteriorly into the posterior commissure and perineal body. Medially the pudendal cleft (*rima pudendi*) lies between them, while laterally they extend to the gluteo-perianal area near the genitofemoral sulcus.

The relatively firm skin corresponds to the scrotum in men and has hairs on the outer aspect. It contains sebaceous glands, sweat glands, and scent glands. A network of smooth muscle fibres can be found in the dermis. The medial aspect is hairless and forms the interlabial fold to the labia minora.

Abundant fatty tissue lying beneath the labia majora affords mechanical protection for the external genital area but also covers the labia minora and helps to close the vaginal vestibule.

Fat atrophy means a loss or at least a reduction of these functions and the outer labia can start to sag. And, like the scrotum, the skin may stretch with age and lead to enlargement (hypertrophy) of the labia majora (Fig. 3).

Labia Minora (Nymphae)

The labia minora (inner labia, inner vaginal lips) are two narrow flaps of the skin that differ widely in shape and size from woman to woman. Ideally they should be completely covered by the labia majora. Their function is to close the vaginal opening to protect against infection and prevent the vagina from drying out.

They run downwards between the labia majora from the mons pubis to the perineum. Proximal to the clitoris, they cover the clitoral shaft (clitoral body), which arches outwards like a half cylinder. This proximal segment forms the clitoral prepuce. The distal part of the prepuce in turn forms an almost circular fold of the skin that closely drapes the glans of the clitoris and is known as the clitoral hood. There is great variation in the shape and length of the clitoral hood. Sometimes it covers only the proximal part of the glans, and sometimes it covers the entire glans, hanging over it like a curtain. The cavity formed between the glans and the inner side of the clitoral hood is called the preputial chamber. Sebaceous glands colonise the neck of

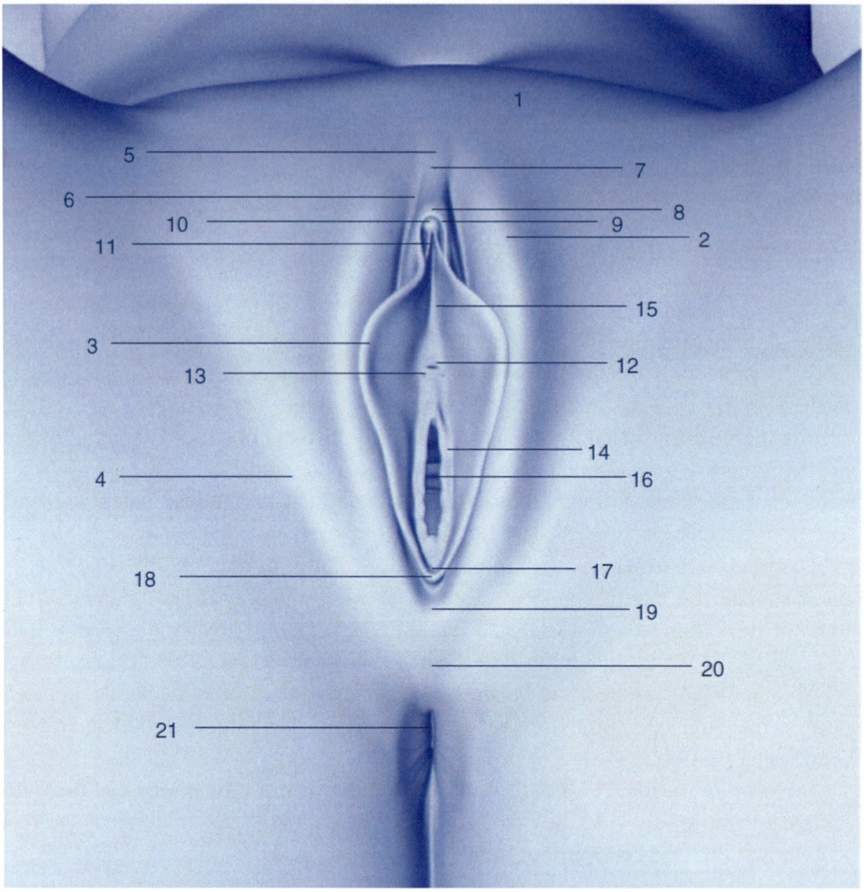

1 mons pubis
2 labia majora
3 labia minora
4 genitofemoral sulcus
5 anterior commissure
6 interlabial fold
7 prepuce, clitoral shaft
8 clitoral hood
9 arch of the clitoral hood
10 glans clitoris
11 frenulum of the clitoris
12 external urethral orifice
13 orifice of the paraurethral glands
14 hymen
15 vaginal vestibule
16 vaginal entry
17 navicular fossa
18 posterior fourchette
19 posterior commissure
20 perineum
21 anus

Fig. 2 Vulva

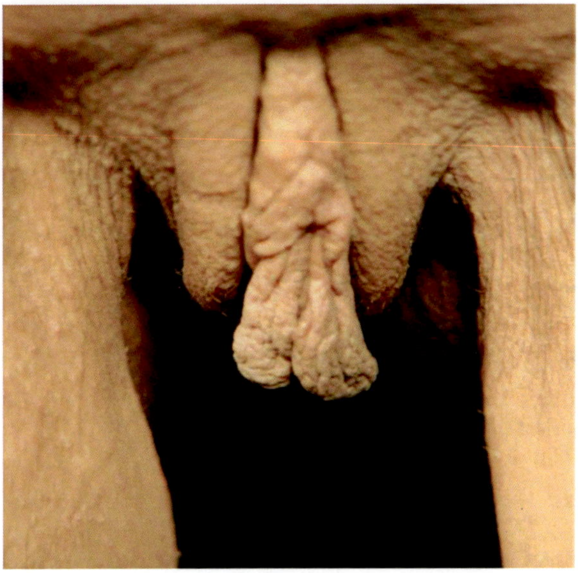

Fig. 3 Ageing appearance of external female genitalia

the glans and produce sebum and smegma, which commonly collect in the preputial chamber. With advancing age, the clitoral hood tends to descend. The lateral parts of the clitoral hood merge into the labia minora surrounding the glans. Sometimes there is a smooth transition at this junction and at other times a distinct step.

The labia minora continue to run downwards along both sides of the vaginal vestibule to the posterior commissure and perineum, where they meet in a bridge of the skin, the frenulum of the labia minora (posterior fourchette).

The height of the labia is greatest immediately below the clitoris. It becomes less as the labia run inferiorly. Distal extensions of the labia minora can radiate across the fourchette along the raphe as far as the anus and merge into the anal skin.

The skin of the inner labia is considerably thinner than that of the outer labia. It is hairless. Morphologically, it is the equivalent of the skin of the penis, or prepuce, in the male. It does not contain any fatty tissue. The inner aspect is covered with vaginal skin (non-keratinised stratified squamous epithelium); the outer aspect is covered with moderately keratinised squamous epithelium. The junction where these two surfaces meet, at the free edges of the labium minora, is known as *Hart's line*.

A layer of loose connective tissue of varying thickness, depending on how thick the labia are, lies between the inner and outer aspects of the labia minora. This layer contains waves of collagen fibres and an abundance of blood vessels and nerves. It represents the subcutaneous "filling material" of the whole external genitalia, likewise surrounding the entire clitoral area and the clitoral shaft (Fig. 4).

With increasing age, but even in young women, the inner labia can grow excessively and protrude beyond the shelter of the outer labia. Apart from the unaesthetic appearance, this may result in functional impairment.

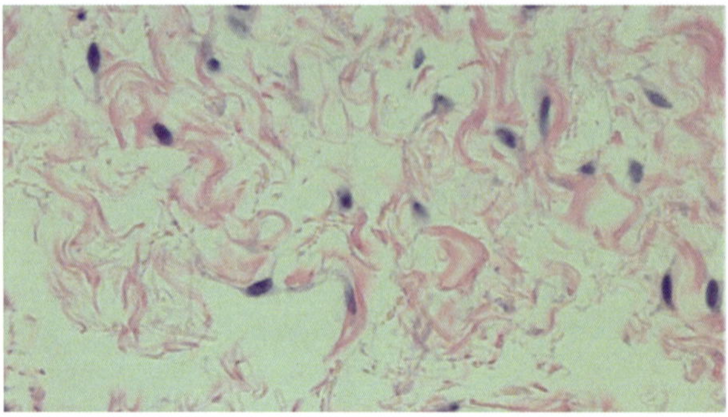

Fig. 4 Subcutaneous tissue

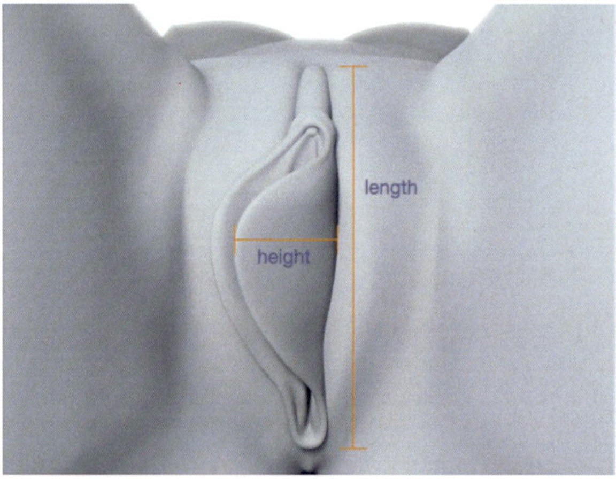

Fig. 5 Labial height and labial length

Although it is often measured differently, the *labia minora length* is the maximum distance from the origin of the labia at the start of the interlabial fold until their insertion into the perineum. The *labia minora height*, on the other hand, is the maximum distance from the base of the interlabial fold to the free edge of the labium minus. This distance is best measured with the patient standing (Fig. 5).

At what point do we refer to hypertrophy of the labia minora? There is no internationally recognised definition. If the labia minora height exceeds 2 cm from the base at the interlabial fold, the inner vaginal lips generally start to be visible outside the shelter of the labia majora and are then associated with more detrimental physical and psychological effects. If they measure more than 2 cm in height, therefore, the labia minora can be described as hypertrophic.

Clitoris

The clitoris is the only organ in the human body that serves exclusively for sexual pleasure. It is a three-dimensional structure in the shape of an inverted Y, the

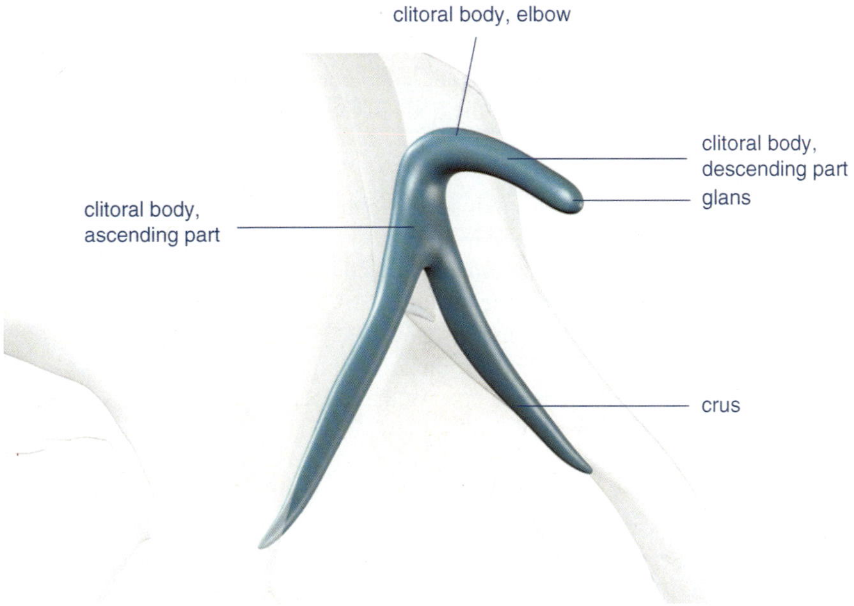

Fig. 6 Clitoris

homologue of the corpora cavernosa of the penis. It consists of two crura that join in the symphyseal midline to form the clitoral body, which then ascends before reversing direction at the elbow to continue downwards. The body is held by the suspensory ligament of the clitoris, which fixes it to the pubic symphysis. The tip of the clitoral shaft, the glans, is the only part of the clitoris that is visible externally (Fig. 6).

Crura

The slightly curved crura (roots) of the clitoris start on the inferior rami of the pubis and the ischium, covered by the ischiocavernosus muscle, which also originates from the rami of the ischium. The crura lie on the inner sides of the pubic and the ischial rami but project beyond the level of the bony margin. They lie below (inferior to) the urogenital diaphragm. At the start, the crura are narrow but increase in thickness as they ascend towards the symphysis. They are about 30–35 mm long, with a mean diameter of about 9 mm (DI MARINO). Their firm consistency is thanks to the surrounding fibroelastic sheath, the tunica albuginea. Histologically, the elements of the clitoris consist of fibroelastic, sponge-like tissue filled with venous sinuses, the corpora cavernosa, which have an erectile potential, as in men. Each corpus cavernosum is supplied with blood by a branch of the superficial perineal artery.

The two crura then run medially and superiorly, following the line of the lower edge of the pubic rami, and continue over the anterior aspect of the symphysis, where they meet in the midline at an angle of about 85°. The section of the clitoris where the two crura meet is called the body of the clitoris.

Body

The body of the clitoris can be subdivided into an ascending part, a curved segment (elbow), and a descending part (Di MARINO).

Fusion of the crura in a superomedial direction gives the ascending part of the clitoral body a triangular shape, measuring up to 2 cm in length, and this lies firmly on the anterior aspect of the symphysis.

Behind it, i.e. between the back of the ascending clitoral body and the symphyseal fascia, is the connective tissue layer of the retrocrural fascia. This fascia covers nerves (dorsal nerve of the clitoris) and blood vessels (dorsal artery of the clitoris) before they reach the cavernous structures.

The apex of the triangular ascending clitoral body lies in the symphyseal midline; its level varies but is usually in the middle-upper third of the anterior surface of the symphysis. This is the point where the crura join. The corpora cavernosa do not amalgamate into a single unit. Together they form a thickened structure, within which they remain separated by a tunica albuginea derived from the fusion of the medial aspects of the tunica covering each crus. A further tunica albuginea then surrounds both corpora cavernosa.

At the apex the clitoris then suddenly changes direction, turning inferiorly in the sagittal plane. This curved part of the clitoral body is known as the elbow. The suspensory ligament of the clitoris, a fascial band, is attached to the tip of this structure: it fixes the body of the clitoris to the pubic symphysis and merges into the tunica albuginea. The section running inferiorly from the elbow is the descending part of the clitoral body, also referred to as the clitoral shaft. It measures approximately 1.5–3 cm in length. The shaft tapers distally to a diameter of about 8 mm.

The glans of the clitoris is found at the end of the shaft. It is the only visible part of the clitoris and is often described as being the size and shape of a pea.

Glans

The glans of the clitoris is the only part of the clitoris that is visible and is erroneously referred to in lay terms as "the clitoris". It has a firm elastic consistency. It is slightly oval in shape, being about 8 mm long and 5 mm wide on average. The skin of the glans is covered by non-keratinised squamous epithelium. At the transition between the glans and clitoral shaft, the proximal part of the glans is known as the clitoral neck. The clitoral hood originates here. A corona, such as is found on the male penis, is rare and usually only very small even when present. Two skinfolds, the frenula of the clitoris, run from below into the distal part of the glans. They are extensions of the labia minora and connected to them in very different ways. Sometimes there is a step at the junction, sometimes there is a smooth transition into the labia minora, and sometimes the frenula even form the main free edges of the labia minora in the distal segment.

The glans consists of spongy tissue without any erectile potential, since the corpora cavernosa do not extend into the glans, even though the septum separating the corpora cavernosa in the descending part of the clitoral body does extend into the proximal part of the glans. The glans has a high density of sensory receptors, especially Pacinian corpuscles, which respond to deep pressure and also sense vibration.

Vestibular Bulb (Corpus Spongiosum)

The vestibular bulbs (corpora spongiosa) comprise dense venous networks that lie above of the Colles fascia in the superficial perineal region below the urogenital diaphragm, on both sides of the urethra, and at the roots of the labia minora on either side of the vaginal vestibule. They flank the "urethrovaginal pyramid" and become thickened and club-shaped inferiorly.

In the midline, the vestibular bulbs communicate through fine veins.

The junction of the two corpora spongiosa below the clitoral body is known as the *pars intermedia* and was described by KÖBELT, as early as 1851 in his book *De l'appareil du sens genital des deux sexes* [On the genital sensory apparatus of the two sexes], as a network of two rows of sinusoidal veins running vertically beneath the clitoral shaft.

In terms of embryonic development, the vestibular bulb in the female corresponds to the corpus spongiosum of the penis, filling with blood during sexual stimulation but without any erectile potential. Each bulb is surrounded by the bulbospongiosus muscle.

According to Di Marino and Lepidi, the corpora cavernosa and corpora spongiosa belong together as components of a single structure that they call the bulbo-clitoral organ.

The vestibular bulbs show considerable variations in length (approximately 3 cm long) and thickness (between 3 and 11 mm thick), depending on how full of blood they are. At the distal end, they may reach as far as the Bartholin's glands.

Vaginal Vestibule

The vaginal vestibule is bordered by the labia minora laterally, the glans clitoris anteriorly, and the frenulum of the labia minora (the fourchette) or extensions of labia majora posteriorly. The vagina, urethra, Bartholin's glands, and paraurethral ducts (Skene's ducts) all open into the vaginal vestibule. The vaginal opening (introitus) is surrounded by the hymen, an almost complete ring of membrane that extends from below the urethral orifice to the vestibular fossa (navicular fossa). The vestibular fossa is an almond-shaped depression between the lower part of the hymen and the fourchette. Anatomically speaking, the hymenal ring demarcates the border between the internal and external genitalia.

Urinary Meatus

The urinary meatus (external urethral orifice) is a slit or a star-shaped structure, which sometimes even forms a papilla. Beyond it lies the urethra, measuring some 2.5–4 cm in length. The urethra extends from the floor of the bladder, passes through the urogenital diaphragm in a slightly concave arch between the symphysis and anterior vaginal wall, and terminates in the external meatus closely beneath the arch of the pubic symphysis.

Greater Vestibular Glands (*Bartholin*'s Glands)

The Bartholin's glands lie on either side at the posterior ends of the vestibular bulbs, embedded in the deep transverse perineal muscle. The ducts open into the vaginal vestibule through orifices about a millimetre in size, situated at the insertion of the labia minora. The mucous secretions moisten the epithelium of the vaginal vestibule.

Lesser Vestibular Glands, Paraurethral Glands (*Skene*'s Glands)

The Skene's glands (named after Alexander Skene (1838–1900), the Scottish gynaecologist who first described them) are tubular mucous glands with multiple ducts opening on either side of the urinary meatus. Their secretions are similar in composition and enzyme pattern to the secretions of the male prostate. This secretion is released in bursts with sexual stimulation or during orgasm, a phenomenon known as female ejaculation or "squirting".

Mons Pubis

The mons pubis extends between the lower abdomen and the origin of the labia majora, covering the pubic symphysis and reaching the inguinal folds laterally. It is a rounded mass of subcutaneous fatty tissue. The start of the pudendal cleft or the superior part of the clitoral shaft can be seen in the midline below the mons pubis. The skin of the mons pubis is relatively thick and hairy. The volume, and therefore the size, of the mons pubis increases in obesity; descent of the mons pubis may occur with age, especially in obese people.

Innervation of the External Genital Area and the Clitoris

The cardinal structure of the sensory innervation of the perineum and the external genital area is the pudendal nerve ("shameful nerve") arising from the end of the spinal cord, together with its terminal branches, in particular, the dorsal nerve of the clitoris.

Amongst other things, it is responsible for sexual stimulation and the ability to experience orgasm. Injury to the nerve may cause irreparable impairment of sensation and stimulation.

The pudendal nerve is the lowest branch of the sacral plexus (S2–S4), which passes through the greater sciatic foramen and runs across the posterior aspect of the ischial spine to return to the pelvis via the lesser sciatic foramen. It then runs with the pudendal artery and vein in the pudendal canal (*Alcock's canal*), in the ischio-anal fossa between the internal obturator muscle and levator ani muscle, covered by the fascia of the internal obturator muscle.

When entering the pudendal canal, the pudendal nerve gives off the inferior rectal nerves, which supply the anal skin and the external anal sphincter muscle.

On leaving the canal, the pudendal nerve branches to give the perineal nerve, which runs medially beneath the urogenital diaphragm, accompanied by the perineal artery.

The superficial branches, the superficial perineal nerves, pass through the superficial perineal fascia (Colles' fascia) to supply the skin of the perineum as sensory nerves and then, as the posterior labial nerves, supply the posterior part of the labia majora, the external orifice of the urethra (urinary meatus), and a large part of the labia minora, especially distal to the clitoris. The deep branches, the deep perineal nerves, are motor nerves that innervate the bulbospongiosus, ischiocavernosus, and external anal sphincter muscles, with sensory components supplying the greater vestibular glands, the corpora spongiosa, and parts of the vaginal vestibule.

Sensory innervation of the anterior third of the labia majora comes mainly from the ilioinguinal nerve (L1), whose terminal branches radiate into the labial skin as the anterior labial nerves. The clitoral hood, the frenula of the clitoris, the labia minora, and the inside of the vaginal vestibule are innervated by the dorsal nerve of the clitoris.

The anterior cutaneous branch of the iliohypogastric nerve, branches of the genitofemoral nerve, and branches of the ilioinguinal nerve provide the sensory supply of the mons pubis (Fig. 7).

After the pudendal canal, the dorsal nerve of the clitoris continues as the terminal branch of the pudendal nerve.

Dorsal Nerve of the Clitoris

The dorsal nerve of the clitoris runs together with the dorsal artery of the clitoris along the lower margin of the inferior pubic ramus, covered by the internal obturator fascia and superior to the urogenital diaphragm. At the inferior margin of the pubic ramus transition to the body of the pubis, i.e. once again out of Alcock's canal, the nerve crosses the dorsal artery of the clitoris, which then lies medial to the nerve. Both these structures penetrate the urogenital diaphragm about 2.7 cm lateral to the urinary meatus (A. VAZE). The dorsal nerve of the clitoris then runs together with the artery across the lower edge of the body of the pubis, in front of the transverse perineal ligament (Krause ligament) at the inferolateral aspect of the pubic arch,

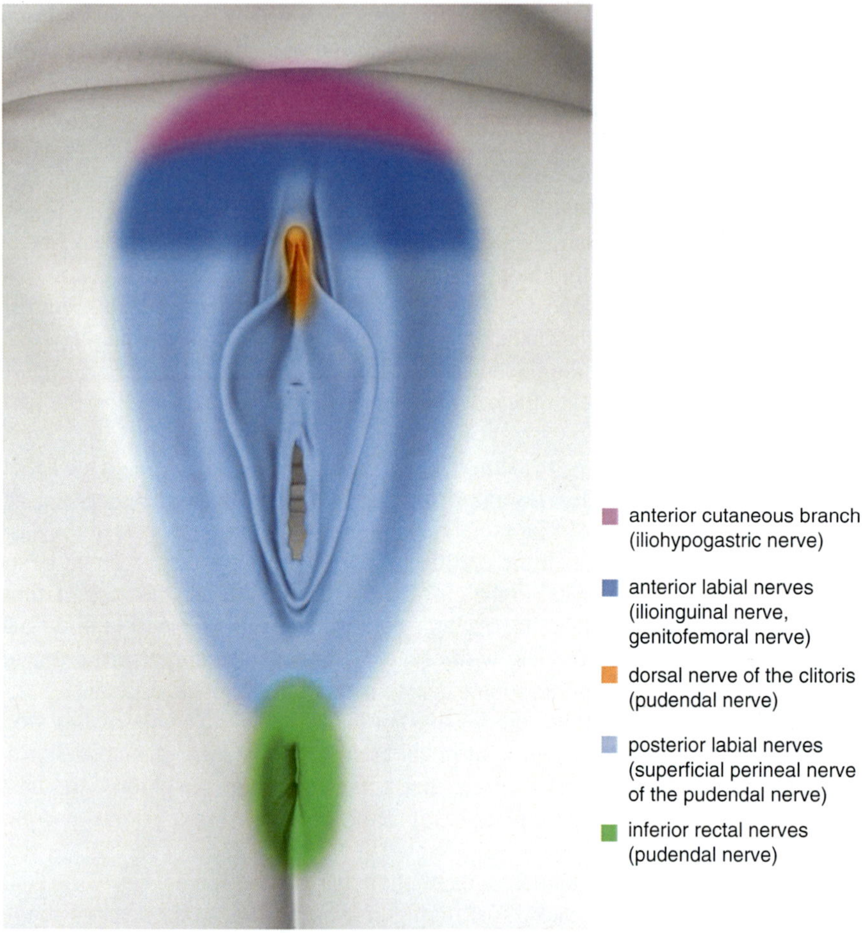

Fig. 7 Sensory innervation pattern of the vulva

covered and protected by parts of the arcuate ligament. The nerve and artery run in close contact with the bone, passing closely over the anterior surface of the ramus and body of the pubis in a superomedial direction in the sulcus nervi dorsalis clitoridis, which is approximately 2.4 mm wide and 16 mm long, to reach the dorsum of the clitoral body. In length, this sulcus spans about 50% of the width of the symphysis in the craniocaudal plane (SEDY). In the sulcus, the nerve and artery are covered by a protective fascia.

Ascending over the anterior aspect of the symphysis, the dorsal nerve of the clitoris unites with the cavernous nerve before reaching the elbow of the clitoris; at this point it can reach a diameter of 2 mm and more (Fig. 8).

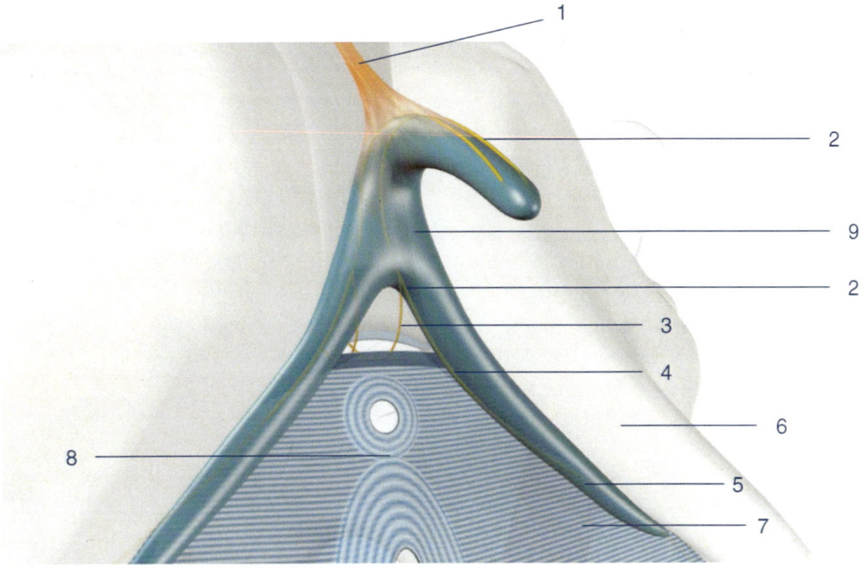

1 suspensory lig. of the clitoris
2 dorsal nerve of the clitoris
3 cavernous nerve of the clitoris
4 pudendal nerve
5 pudendal canal (*Alcock* canal)
6 inferior pubic ramus
7 urogenital diaphragm
8 urethrovaginal m.
9 clitoris

Fig. 8 Dorsal nerve of the clitoris

This fusion turns the dorsal nerve of the clitoris into a mixed nerve with both cerebrospinal and autonomic components: it supplies sensory function to the glans, the clitoral hood, and the corpora cavernosa, motor function to the deep transverse muscles and the external urethral sphincter, and autonomic function to the corpora cavernosa and spongiosa (Di MARINO).

The right and left dorsal nerves of the clitoris lie about 5–10 mm from each other. The slightly medial path of the nerve now changes to a vertical course, and together with the dorsal artery of the clitoris, it pierces the retrocrural fascia to enter the retrocrural space (Fig. 9). The dorsal vein joins them medially (not illustrated here).

The nerve runs on the dorsum of the clitoral body, along the angle of the elbow, penetrates the deep component of the suspensory ligament, and continues on the

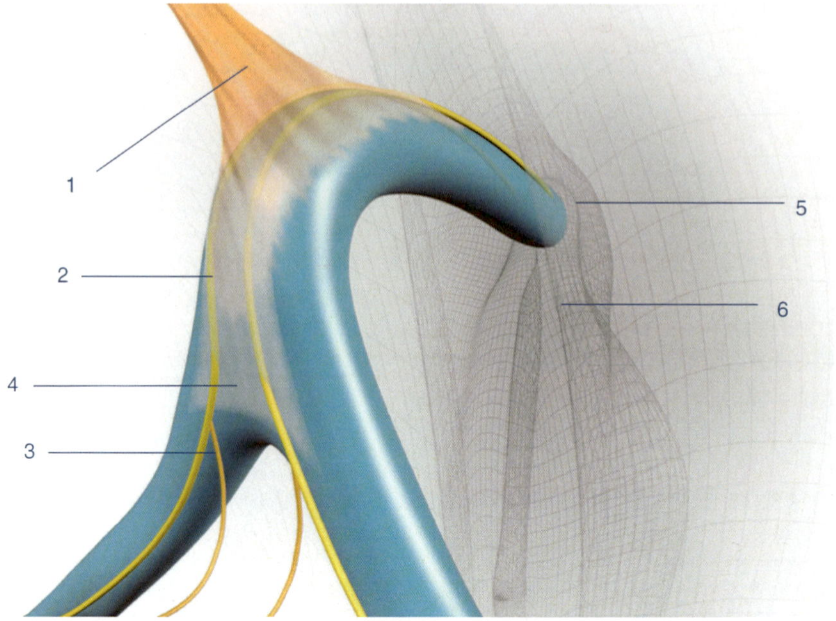

1 suspensory lig. of the clitoris
2 dorsal nerve of the clitoris
3 cavernous nerve of the clitoris
4 retrocrural fascia
5 clitoral hood
6 labia minora

Fig. 9 Dorsal nerve of the clitoris, cavernous nerve of the clitoris penetrating the retrocrural fascia

clitoral shaft, beneath the clitoral fascia at the 11 o'clock or 1 o'clock position, close to the tunica albuginea; it then runs distally along the descending part of the clitoris towards the glans. The dorsal artery of the clitoris lies medial to the nerve and even further medially, close to the midline, is the dorsal vein of the clitoris, which does not rest so closely on the tunica albuginea. According to Baskin et al., the nerve is not to be found at the 12 o'clock position.

In its path towards the glans, the nerve largely maintains its size and runs slightly more laterally. It gives off small branches at right angles to its axis and, after passing through the tunica albuginea, also branches to the corpora cavernosa. The small branches extend predominantly to the tactile corpuscles concentrated around the clitoral shaft. Superficial branches of the dorsal nerve of the clitoris also run over the clitoral fascia, i.e. in the subcutaneous space beneath the prepuce.

Slightly proximal to the clitoral hood, the nerve breaks through the tunica albuginea and plunges beneath the corona into the glans. Its terminal branches ramify through the glans, running only just below the surface, and radiate into the genital corpuscles (the sensory receptors located beneath the epithelium). The densest innervation is on the dorsal aspect of the glans.

The terminal branches of the nerve continue over the glans and, as mentioned previously, contribute to the sensory innervation, in particular of the lateral parts of the clitoral hood, the frenulum of the clitoris, the labia minora, the spongy structures, and a considerable part of the lateral wall of the vaginal vestibule.

Cavernous Nerve

The vesical plexuses arise from the inferior hypogastric plexus (pelvic plexus) on each side and spread over both sides of the fundus of the bladder. The autonomic cavernous nerves arise from here. They run downwards in the 10 o'clock and 2 o'clock positions along the anterior wall of the vagina and continue at 7 o'clock and 5 o'clock along the urethra, before running beneath the arcuate ligament to reach the dorsum of the clitoral body. There the cavernous nerve unites with the dorsal nerve of the clitoris on each side. The cavernous nerve is comparatively thin, being only a sixth of the size of the dorsal nerve of the clitoris.

The inferior hypogastric plexus induces parasympathetic mechanisms in the corpora spongiosa and cavernosa via the autonomic fibres of the cavernous nerve, causing the clitoris and the labia to swell with sexual stimulation. Tissue swelling as a result of vasodilatation in turn enhances the tactile resonance of the clitoris and thus augments the sexual response. Injury to the cavernous nerve may thus alter the perfusion dynamics, resulting in a reduced ability to experience orgasm and diminished lubrication of the genital area (Bekker).

In classic anatomy textbooks, we find very little on the precise course of the dorsal nerve of the clitoris after it has pierced the urogenital diaphragm.

In this respect, we need to thank authors such as Helen O'Connell, V. Ginger, and J. Sedy whose work has provided more detailed knowledge in recent years. The book by Vincent Di Marino and Hubert Lepidi, *Anatomic Study of the Clitoris and the Bulbo-Clitoral Organ,* is to be particularly recommended: from every possible point of view, it is a marvellous work on the clitoris and surrounding area.

Vascular Supply

Thanks to the rich vascular supply of the genitalia, we can take a generous approach to tissue perfusion with locoregional tissue transfer. Wounds heal faster than in other areas, as long as there is no early or intense friction. The excellent vascular supply means that wound infection is a rare exception.

The blood supply to the external sex organs comes mainly from the internal pudendal artery. The anterior third of the labia majora and labia minora as well as mons pubis are also supplied with arterial blood from the external iliac artery via the inferior epigastric artery and from the femoral artery via the external pudendal artery and its terminal branches, the anterior labial arteries.

The internal pudendal artery arises from the internal iliac artery and passes out of the ischioanal fossa to the inferior surface of the urogenital diaphragm, giving off the perineal artery medially. The terminal branches of the perineal artery run into the bulbospongiosus and ischiocavernosus muscles and, as the posterior labial arteries, pass through the Colles' fascia into the labia. The transverse perineal artery, also a small branch of the perineal artery, supplies the posterior extensions of the labia and the perineum.

The urethral artery, a short vessel, branches on the urethra and the bulbs and sends branches to supply the bulbs.

The clitoris and the corpus cavernosum are supplied by the clitoral artery (also arising from the internal pudendal artery), which divides along its course into the deep artery of the clitoris (supplying branches into the corpus cavernosum of the clitoris) and the dorsal artery of the clitoris, which lies medial to the accompanying dorsal nerve of the clitoris, and runs along the dorsum of the clitoral shaft to terminate distally in the glans.

The deep dorsal veins of the clitoris lie medial to the dorsal artery of the clitoris and run across the arcuate ligament to drain into the inferior vesical plexus. The superficial dorsal veins of the clitoris run along the clitoral shaft also in the 12 o'clock position, immediately below the skin, and are tributaries of the external pudendal vein.

The veins generally follow the same course as the arterial vessels. In the mid-genital area, they form numerous venous plexuses along the labia and the vestibule and also intravaginally. These plexuses become congested (swell), especially with sexual stimulation.

Patient Evaluation and Preparation

Evaluation

The selection of patients with respect to their suitability for intimate surgery is not very complicated, as long as expectations on the visual and functional outcome largely coincide with surgical feasibility.

The main reasons motivating a woman to undergo surgical correction are problems of a functional and/or aesthetic nature.

Such problems include recurrent intertriginous irritation of the skin, discomfort during sexual intercourse, and rubbing and pain when wearing tight-fitting clothing or during sporting activities such as cycling. The effects of the aesthetically unpleasing appearance often go beyond a simple "I don't like it" to become issues causing an anxiety about sexual encounters that have a negative impact on the woman's sex life and may lead to avoidance of any sexual contact at all, even within a marriage.

There are usually functional and aesthetic components mixed with various psychological aspects. Rarely does a woman simply say she "doesn't like" her appearance without there being some associated physical impairment or psychological problem.

Unlike earlier surveys of our patients, which allowed us to distinguish only between aesthetic and functional impairment, a more discerning questionnaire has now brought us greater insight on the problems. Our results are largely in agreement with the study by Trichot et al. nearly all sexually active women have functional symptoms from invagination of the labia during sexual intercourse, with pain, irritation of the skin and swelling, recurrent fungal infection, deviation of the urine stream and anatomical alterations of the introitus with functional problems such inability to close the vaginal entry, dry vagina with recurrent infections or sexual impairment, irrespective of the fact that the external appearance may also be unacceptable. In addition, there are injuries following vaginal delivery, e.g. from

S. Gress, *Aesthetic and Functional Labiaplasty*,
DOI 10.1007/978-3-319-60222-6_2

episiotomies and, more recently, repairs of previous botched operations. The survey was carried out over the past 3 years (since 2014), with responses from more than 850 of our patients, this large number of cases making it representative.

Preparation

Surgery on the external genitalia can be carried out extremely well under local anaesthetic. Apart from following the usual guidelines prior to any surgical procedure, such as stopping aspirin, etc. for 14 days beforehand, no special preparation is needed for intimate surgery. Patients should be completely shaved in the genital area.

Photodocumentation

Standardised settings for the aperture and shutter speed of the camera (we use a digital single lens reflex with a light-sensitive objective), in addition to standardised lighting conditions, with photographs taken in the same position before and after surgery, are necessary to show the outcome of the procedure as objectively as possible:

The background is blue. The most important positions for the photographs are a frontal view with the patient standing, a lateral oblique view in the lithotomy position, and a frontal view in the lithotomy position. Directly after the procedure, repeat the photographs, at least those in the lithotomy position (Fig. 1a, b).

If possible, take follow-up photographs after 6 months, i.e. when all swelling has completely subsided. Unfortunately, these images are not so easy to obtain, as patients are not always willing to travel the sometimes considerable distance to the practice only for a follow-up examination.

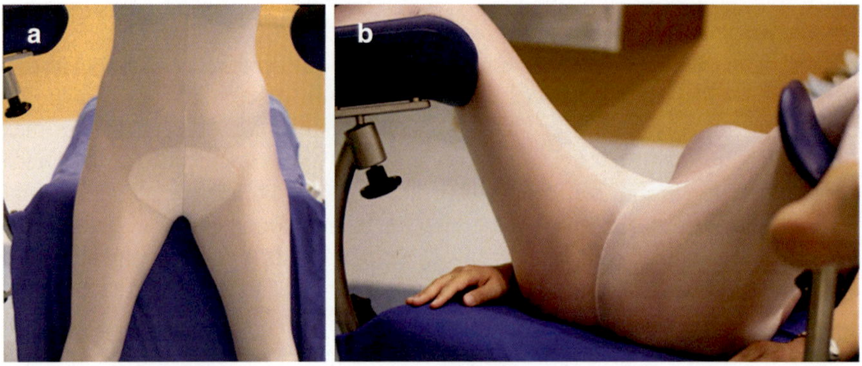

Fig. 1 Photodocumentation from different positions (**a**) frontal view, standing; (**b**) oblique view, lithotomy position

Medication

Adequate analgesia should be prescribed before every surgical procedure, as pain that may last for several days has to be reckoned with, especially after extensive correction of the labia minora and alteration of the position of the clitoris. Peripherally active analgesics may not always be sufficiently effective, so that it is worthwhile combining them with a centrally acting agent. The routine administration of antibiotics is somewhat disputed, but we give cephalosporin as blanket antibiotic cover.

Patient Consent

According to the legal regulations, preoperative briefing sessions should be held in good time before surgery. Patients should be informed of the following aspects and time taken to discuss them:

Swelling

There is always swelling, which usually goes down by 80% after 6 weeks and disappears entirely by 6 months.

Pain

Pain usually lasts up to 3 days after the operation, rarely longer.

Postoperative Bleeding, Haematomas

Postoperative bleeding that requires surgical revision is rare; bruising and small haematomas are possible.

Disorders of Wound Healing

Statistically speaking, this is the most common complication at 4%. Rubbing/friction should therefore be avoided.

Scars

Wounds usually heal without scarring. Painful or pronounced scars are very rare.

Disorders of Sensation

Disorders of sexual sensation are not to be expected if the operation is performed correctly. Transient alterations in sensation along the line of the incision may occur as hypersensitivity or hyposensitivity but return to normal once the wound has healed.

Infection

Infection is rare because of the good tissue perfusion and can be almost ruled out with routine antibiotic prophylaxis.

Asymmetry
Asymmetry is possible following correction of the labia minora, entirely due to a different course of healing in the left and the right sides.

Possible revision operation
Revision may be necessary if there is asymmetry or delayed wound healing.

Dimple Formation
With liposuction

Over−/Undercorrection
For example, with autologous fat transfer to the labia majora (*Lipostructure*), the proportion of non-healing fatty tissue is relatively high.

Outpatient Procedure

Operations on the external genitalia can be carried out quite easily as outpatient procedures, because they are usually performed under local anaesthetic. But an overnight stay in hospital is not normally required, even after a general anaesthetic. It must, however, be ensured that the wound is checked the following day. The patient should also be able to ask any questions or contact the surgeon at any time in an emergency.

Equipment

Marking
Use a fine permanent marker with ink that will not run on moist skin to indicate the resection lines, and toothless forceps to make it easier to mark the resection lines at the same level on the inner and outer aspects of the labia minora (Fig. 2)

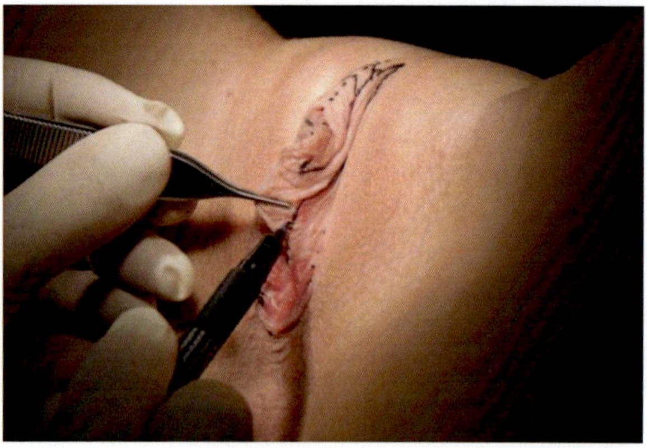

Fig. 2 Forceps facilitates marking

Instruments
1 fine Adson forceps
1 nerve dissection scissors with fine rounded tips
1 needle holder
1 mosquito clip (Fig. 3)

High-Frequency Unit 2.2 MH
This device allows cutting without burning, and also coagulation. Settings of 25–30 W. The skin does not have to be stretched for the incision (Fig. 4)

Operating Table
Adjustable table with the possibility of the lithotomy position.

Lighting
Two operating theatre lamps to illuminate the surgical field without shadows.

Monitoring
Standard monitoring and emergency equipment, e.g. pulse oximeter.

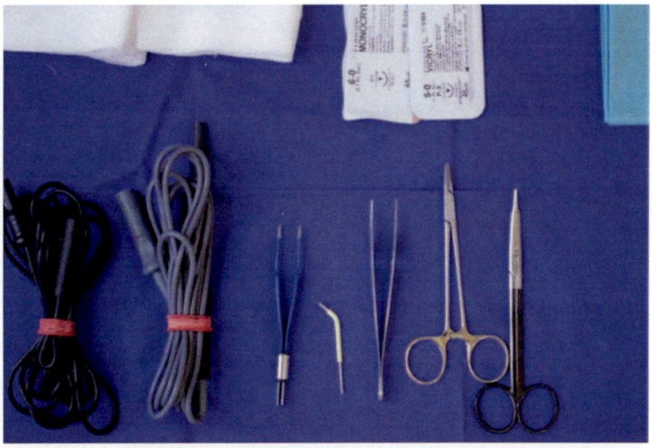

Fig. 3 Instruments for labiaplasty

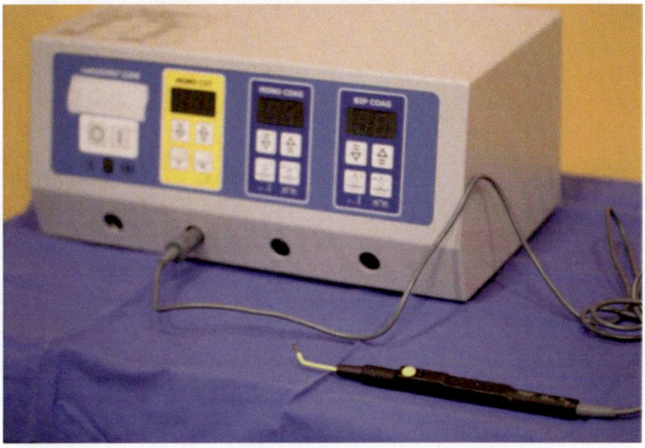

Fig. 4 High-frequency unit

Surgical Goals

Achieving the best possible function with an optimal appearance is of particular significance in female genital surgery: aesthetically unpleasing genitalia can have a negative impact on a woman's sex life.

Unfortunately, not every surgeon is aware of this requirement. From the cosmetic point of view, inappropriate procedures or botched operations can make the situation much worse and cause the patient considerable psychological distress. It goes without saying that maintaining the sensitivity of the area is of prime importance.

Even though there are huge cultural, ethnic, and individual variations in the concept of beauty, there seems to be an image of the vulva that all women in our Western society would consider ideal. It is an image of firm, well-shaped outer labia that completely enclose and cover the inner labia, giving the appearance of a closed shell (Fig. 5).

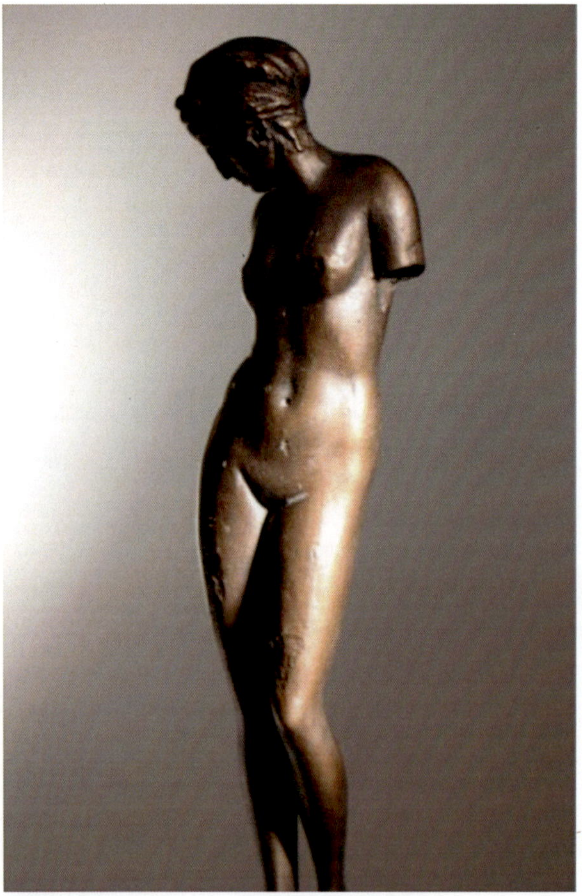

Fig. 5 "The Girl from Beroia", Goddess of Beauty and Love (2./1. century b.c., bronze statuette, Antique State Collection, Glyptothec, Munich)

The shape and size of the individual vulval structures can differ considerably. There is a huge range of variation.

The fullness and consistency of the labia majora not only affect their own appearance, but also determine whether the labia minora are partially or completely covered, and the extent to which these inner lips protrude. Whether or not they are completely enclosed by the outer labia obviously also depends mainly on the labia minora height.

The position, length, and width of the clitoral shaft, together with the size and position of the glans clitoris, are also key factors.

Labia Minora

Ideal Appearance

The ideal appearance of the labia minora is somewhat more varied than that of the labia majora. Some patients want their inner vaginal lips to be as short as possible, while others prefer a longer version, usually gently curved. In most cases, however, the prepuce should lie tightly over the clitoral shaft and the clitoral hood fit firmly over the glans, covering some two-thirds to all of it (Fig. 1).

It is not clear where this concept of the "ideal appearance" has come from, but it is possibly related to pictures posted on the Internet, which are very easily accessed these days.

Anatomical Considerations

For the surgical approach to labia reduction (labiaplasty), it is worth dividing the course of the labia minora into three segments:

Segment 1: Proximal to (above) the clitoris
Segment 2: At the level of the clitoris
Segment 3: Distal to (below) the clitoris (Fig. 2)

The shape and appearance of segments 1 and 2 are decisively influenced by the size and position of the clitoral shaft. Together with the fullness of the labia majora and the shape of the labia minora and the prepuce, these clitoral shaft parameters determine whether the pudendal cleft forms a narrow line or whether the labia minora already visibly protrude from the pudendal cleft at their origin (Fig. 3a, b).

At the end of the clitoral shaft, the position of the glans in its spatial relationship to the anterior plane of the symphysis depends on the angle of the clitoral elbow: if this angle is acute, the clitoral shaft runs more closely to the symphysis, so the glans also lies deeper "inside" and can more easily be covered by the labia majora.

S. Gress, *Aesthetic and Functional Labiaplasty*,
DOI 10.1007/978-3-319-60222-6_3

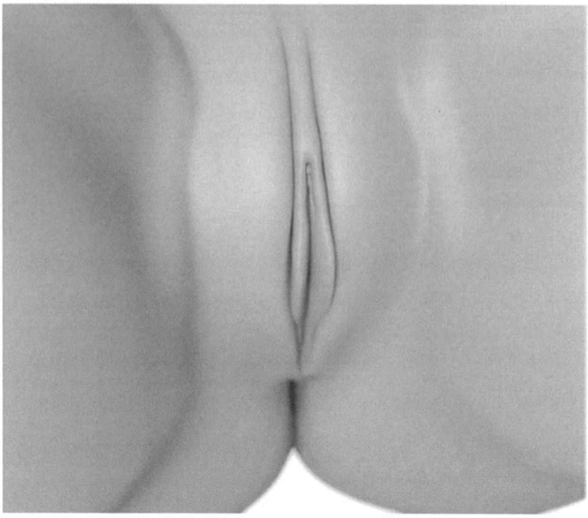

Fig. 1 "Ideal appearance" of the labia minora

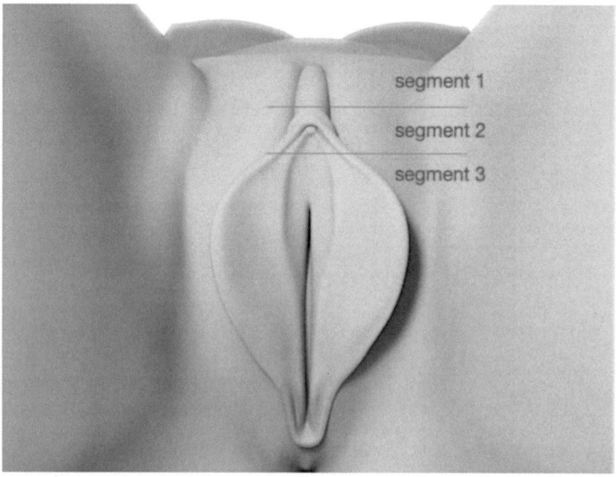

Fig. 2 Subdivision of the labia minora

Conversely, with an obtuse angle of the clitoral elbow, the glans stands further forward and may then be termed "clitoral protrusion" (Fig. 4).

There is considerable variation in the distance found between the glans of the clitoris and the urinary meatus. It can be anything between 1 and 7 cm or more. Interestingly enough, there is a reliable fixed point: the external urethral orifice is always in the midline just beneath the lower edge of the pubic arch. If the distance from this point to the glans differs so greatly from woman to woman, it means that the interval must be determined solely by the variable position and size of the clitoris and its components—the length of the crura, the clitoral shaft, and the glans (Fig. 5).

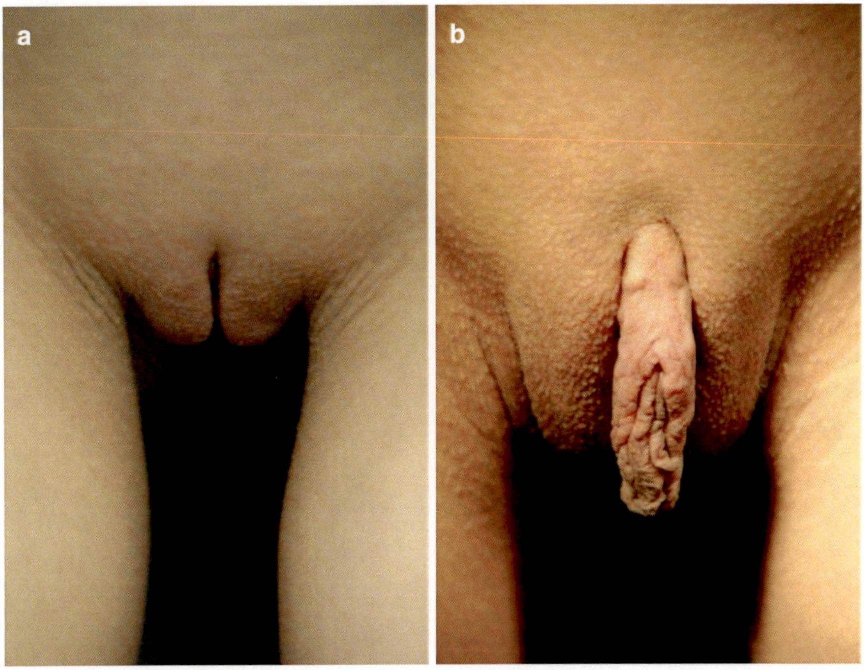

Fig. 3 (**a**) Narrow pudendal cleft. (**b**) Wide pudendal cleft with protruding clitoral shaft and labia minor hypertrophy

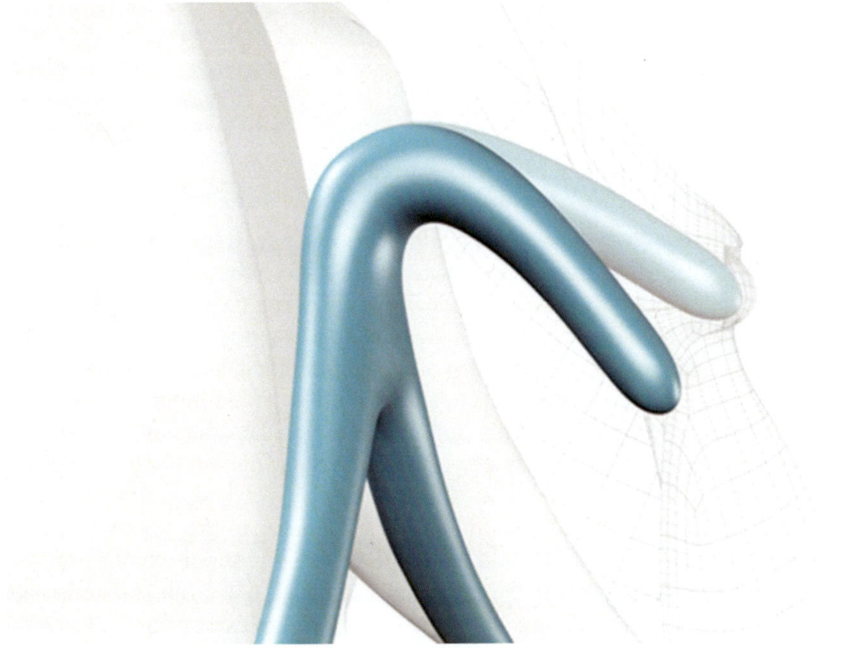

Fig. 4 Relationship between the postition of the clitoral shaft and the angle of the clitoral elbow, lateral view

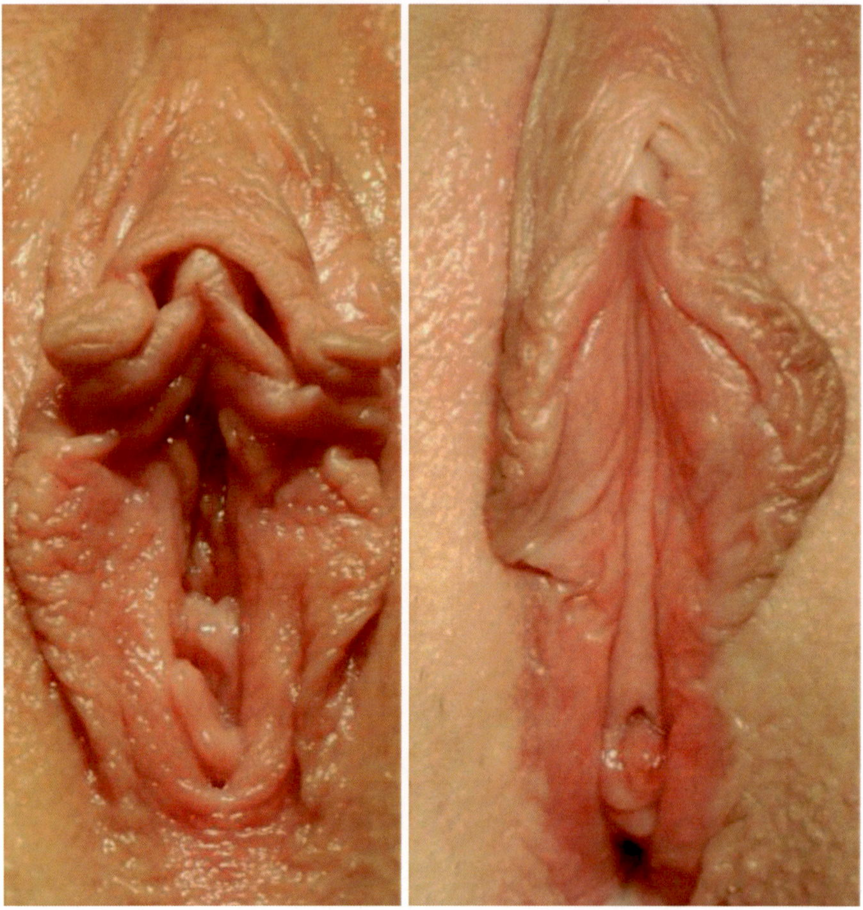

Fig. 5 Short and long distance between urinary meatus and the glans

The clitoral hood varies considerably in size and shape. Hypertrophy of the labia usually also affects the clitoral hood, which can be very pronounced and hang over the glans like a curtain. It is then also clearly visible (Fig. 6a–d).

In size and shape, the glans can be compared to a pea. It is usually completely or almost completely covered by the skin of the clitoral hood, but may sometimes lie completely exposed, although this is not common. The paired frenula radiating into the inferior surfaces of the glans run downwards to join the labia minora. Variations occur here, too: the junction may be very soft, merging smoothly into the labia, or it may show an obvious discontinuity in the line.

The third segment of the labia minora lies inferiorly to the clitoris. The labia continue, surrounding the vaginal vestibule, to the posterior commissure and sometimes even further across the perineum to the anus. As a rule, the inner labia consist of only a single skinfold but sometimes there are two or rarely even more.

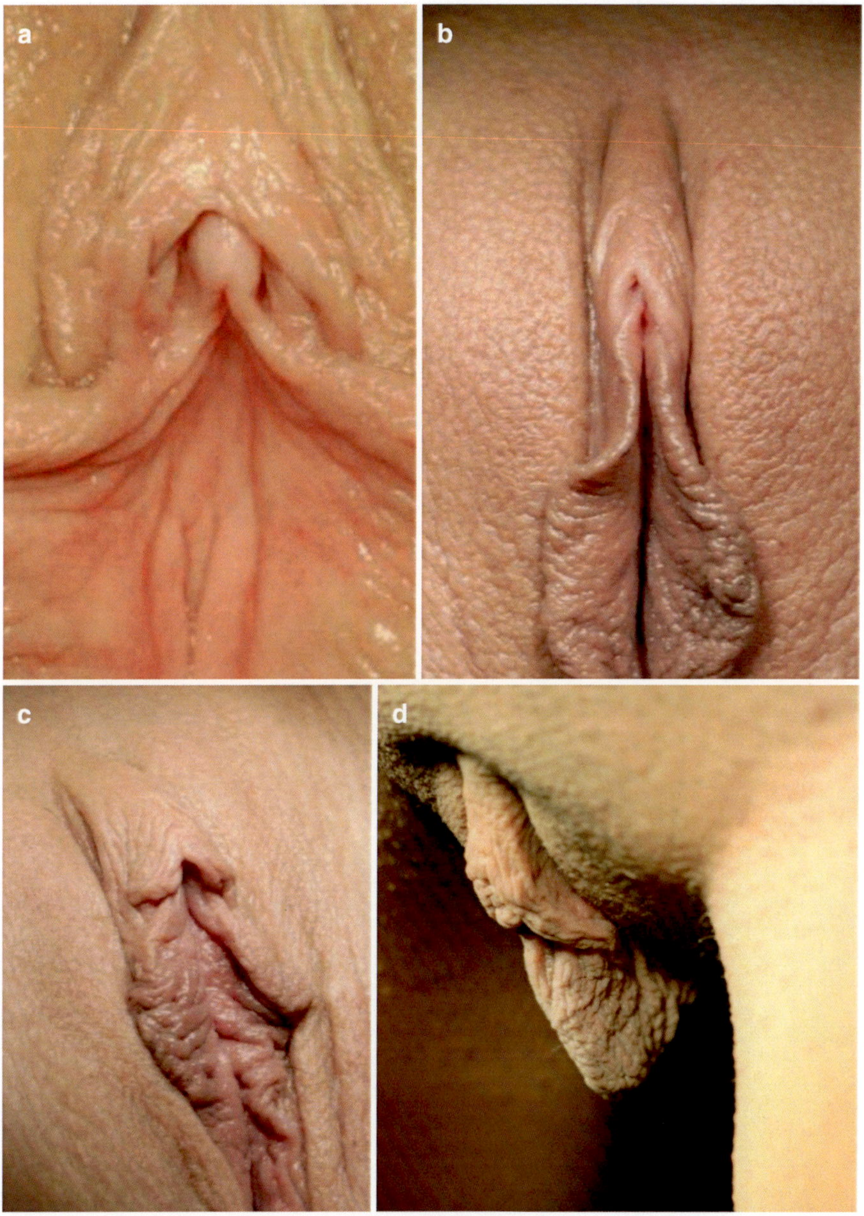

Fig. 6 Variations of the clitoral hood. (**a**) Short clitoral hood exposing the glans; (**b**) Clitoral hood covering the glans; (**c**) Large, hanging clitoral hood; (**d**) Large, hanging clitoral hood; standing position; oblique view

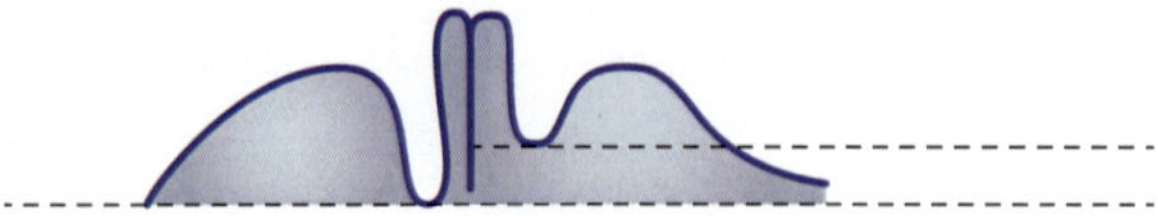

Fig. 7 Different levels of the labial base

The height of the labia minora, measured from the base of the interlabial fold, is greatest immediately below the clitoris and decreases as they run towards the posterior commissure. When there is labial hypertrophy, the labial height can reach a considerable 5 cm or more.

Interestingly enough, the level of the labial base can also vary in relation to the vaginal vestibule. This factor should also be taken into consideration in the preoperative evaluation. A high baseline means that even a small labial height may be enough for the inner labia to protrude from the covering outer labia (Fig. 7).

Labia Minora Reduction (Labiaplasty)

Preparation

Hypertrophy of the labia minora can be operated on under local anaesthetic without problem. The patient's genital area should be completely shaved. It is worth administering a peripherally acting analgesic immediately before the procedure and giving routine infection prophylaxis with a broad-spectrum antibiotic. Taking preoperative photographs during the preparation is also to be recommended: one with the patient standing and then frontal and lateral views in the lithotomy position. The patient remains in the lithotomy position throughout the operation. Make sure that the back and buttocks are adequately cushioned, as otherwise problems may arise from the relatively long time that the patient will be lying on her back. For safety reasons, insert a peripheral venous access, and monitor the pulse rate and oxygen saturation with a pulse oximeter. Disinfect the genital area with a mucosal disinfectant. Mark out the incision lines once the disinfectant has dried.

Markings

Irrespective of how pronounced the findings are, the main decision is how much tissue is to be left and not how much is to be removed. This is the main focus of consideration. When in doubt, it is better to remove a little less tissue than to remove too much, as the skin will shrink somewhat after the operation.

Mark the incision lines *before* injecting the local anaesthetic; otherwise a reliable assessment of the anatomy will no longer be possible because of tissue swelling. So as not to confuse incision lines with lines made for orientation purposes, it is a good idea to use different colours or differently constructed lines, e.g. dotted lines or dashes (Fig. 8).

Always mark the midline along the clitoral shaft and the interlabial folds first, to use for orientation. The definitive incision lines can then be drawn in depending on the technique to be used in each case. A fine toothless Adson forceps is helpful to mark the outer and inner aspects of the labia minora at the same level on each surface.

If the patient so wishes, you can show her the markings and incision lines with the aid of a hand mirror and explain how much of the labia will be removed and just how much left. Any necessary adjustments can then be made promptly.

Anaesthetic

When they have decided on a local anaesthetic, all patients are somewhat anxious about the injection. Reports and tales published on the Internet are partly responsible for their fears. When you get to this stage in the proceedings, take enough time to make sure that the atmosphere in the operating room is as quiet and relaxed as possible. It is often comforting for the patient to hold the nurse's hand during the injection.

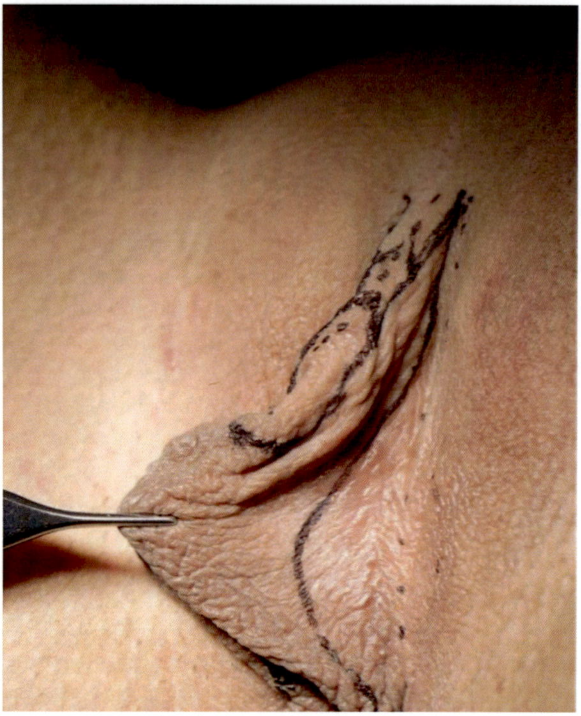

Fig. 8 Uninterrupted lines mark the lines of incision

For labia minora reductions, we use about 10 ml 1% lidocaine with added adrenaline at a concentration of 1:100,000. Give the injection through a very fine, 27-gauge (0.4 mm) needle with a length of 40 mm.

Start the injection on the inner aspect of the labia minora, as this is less painful than through the outer skin. From here, the whole area can be reached easily, especially the clitoral shaft and the dorsal nerve of the clitoris, and distally the base of the labia minora in the interlabial fold to the posterior commissure and even further to the anus. A pudendal block is not necessary, but the area has to be infiltrated with the added adrenaline to keep the perioperative bleeding to a minimum (Fig. 9).

When surgery is carried out under a general anaesthetic, the area is still injected with lidocaine and adrenaline, to reduce bleeding and maintain an even general anaesthesia.

Techniques

One feature common to the techniques I am about to describe is that they all bring about a reduction in the whole length of the labia minora, from the origin at the mons pubis to the insertion into the perineum, and do not treat only the part distal to the clitoris. The methods differ in a few details, depending on the extent of the anatomical findings and the corrective measures consequently required.

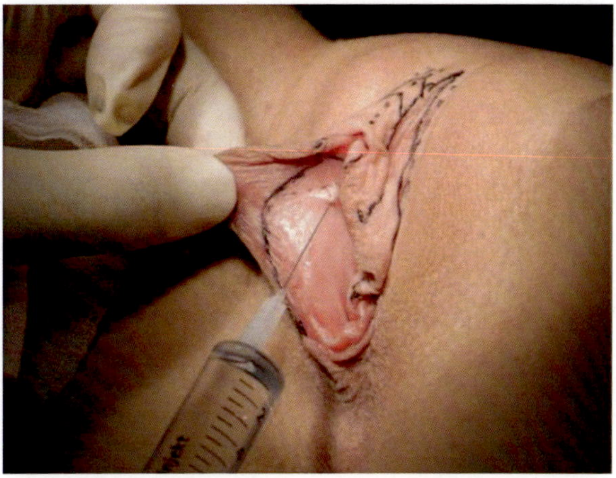

Fig. 9 Infiltration of local anaesthetics

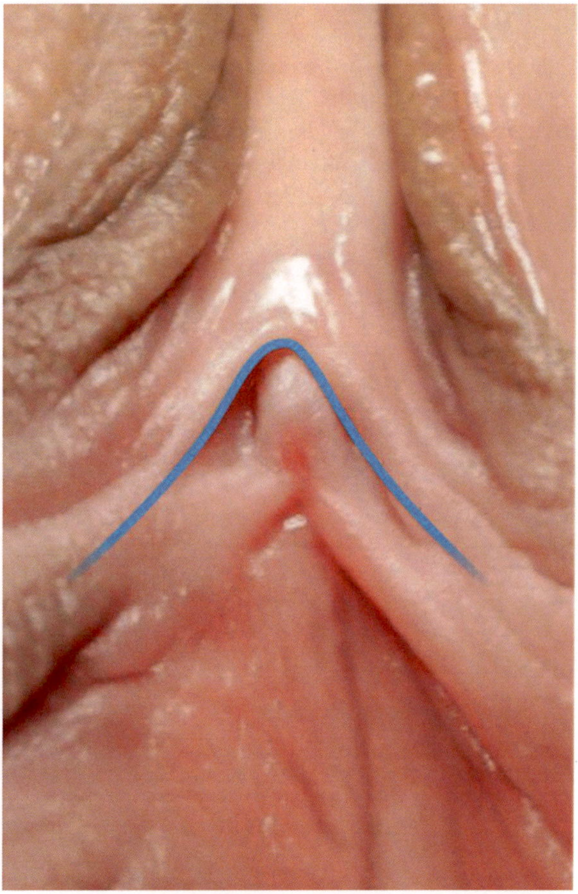

Fig. 10 Disruption of the arch of the clitoral hood (*blue line*) should be avoided

"Composite reduction labiaplasty" is the technique that meets all conceivable requirements and, in my opinion, can be considered the maximum variant of the feasible and the possible. For this reason, this method is described down to the smallest detail. All preoperative preparation, suture materials, and suturing techniques are the same for all the following procedures.

It shall be emphasised that none of these techniques interrupts or disrupts the integrity of the arch of the clitoral hood in any way. And this integrity should not be disrupted, as it is hardly possible to restore it in a natural way. In exceptional cases, e.g. with a troublesome exposed clitoris, this arch can be removed and the inner aspects of the clitoral hood fixed together in the midline so as to maintain a covering for the clitoris. As a rule, if the natural rounded curve of the arch of the clitoral hood is lost in the process, it is extremely difficult to restore (Fig. 10).

Composite Reduction Labiaplasty (CRL)

As its name indicates, the resection in this method creates completely separate labial segments, and these are then combined to give a uniform whole with the desired aesthetic results. When the individual segments are joined together, there is a degree of superior and inferior tension with optimal tightening of the labia minora and the clitoral hood along their entire length (Fig. 11).

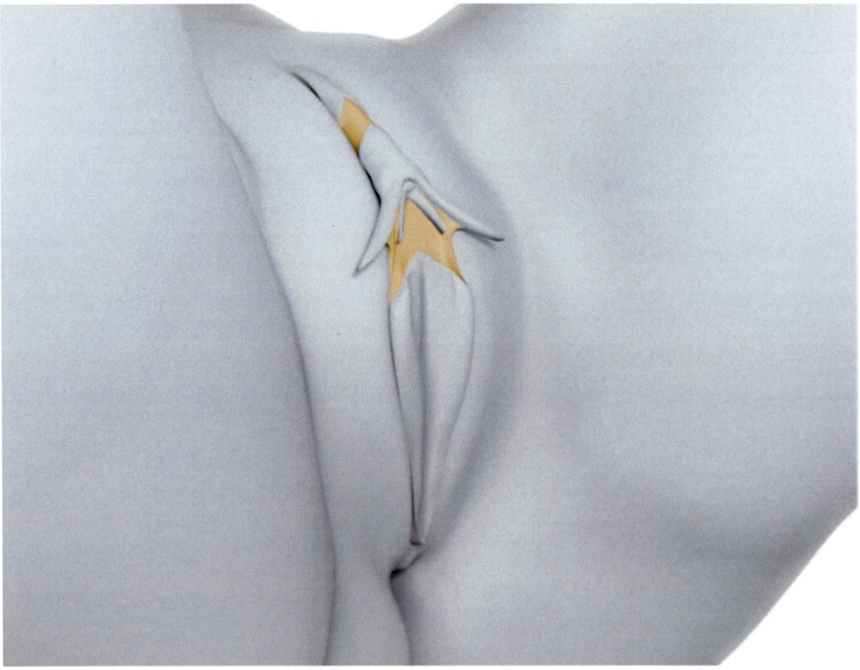

Fig. 11 Three separate labial segments created by the composite reduction labiaplasty

Indication

This method is suitable for hypertrophy of the labia minora in all three segments, i.e. above the clitoris and the prepuce, at the level of the clitoris with the clitoral hood, and below the clitoris. This procedure is the method of choice to lift the clitoral hood and shorten the prepuce, to give the appearance of shortening the clitoral shaft, and to correct any clitoral protrusion (Fig. 12).

Operation

The incision starts at the posterior commissure or at the posterior fourchette and runs upwards. In this way, any bleeding will not obstruct the view of the markings (Fig. 13).

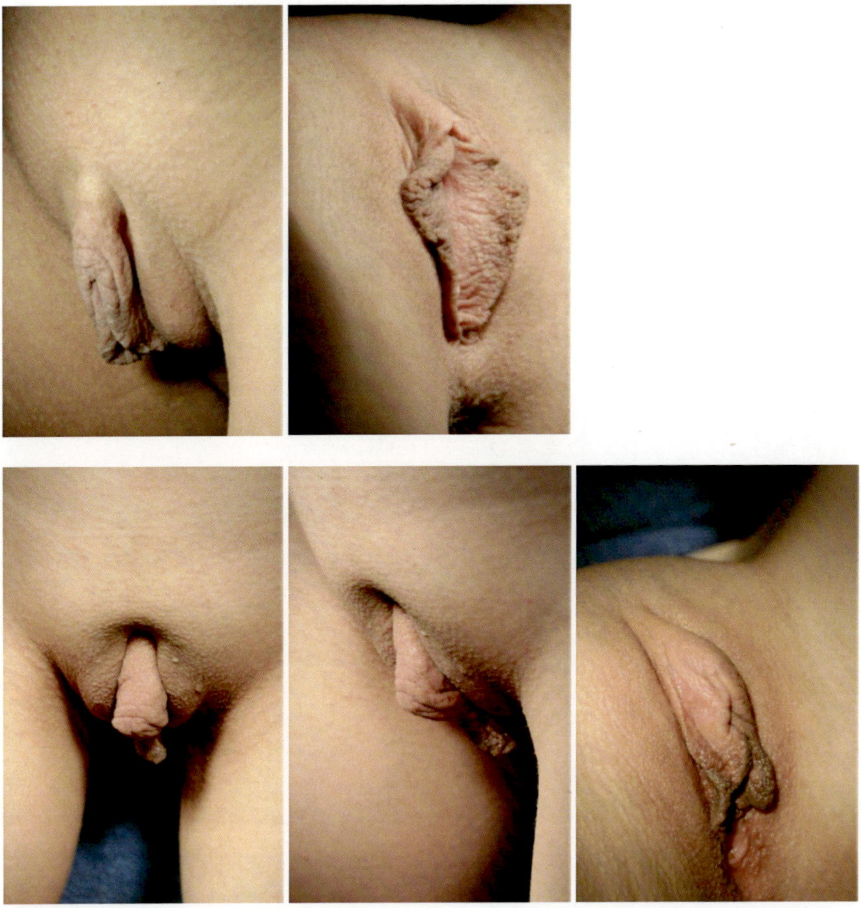

Fig. 12 Patients with labia hypertrophy in all segments; large, hanging clitoral hood; clitoral protrusion in different views

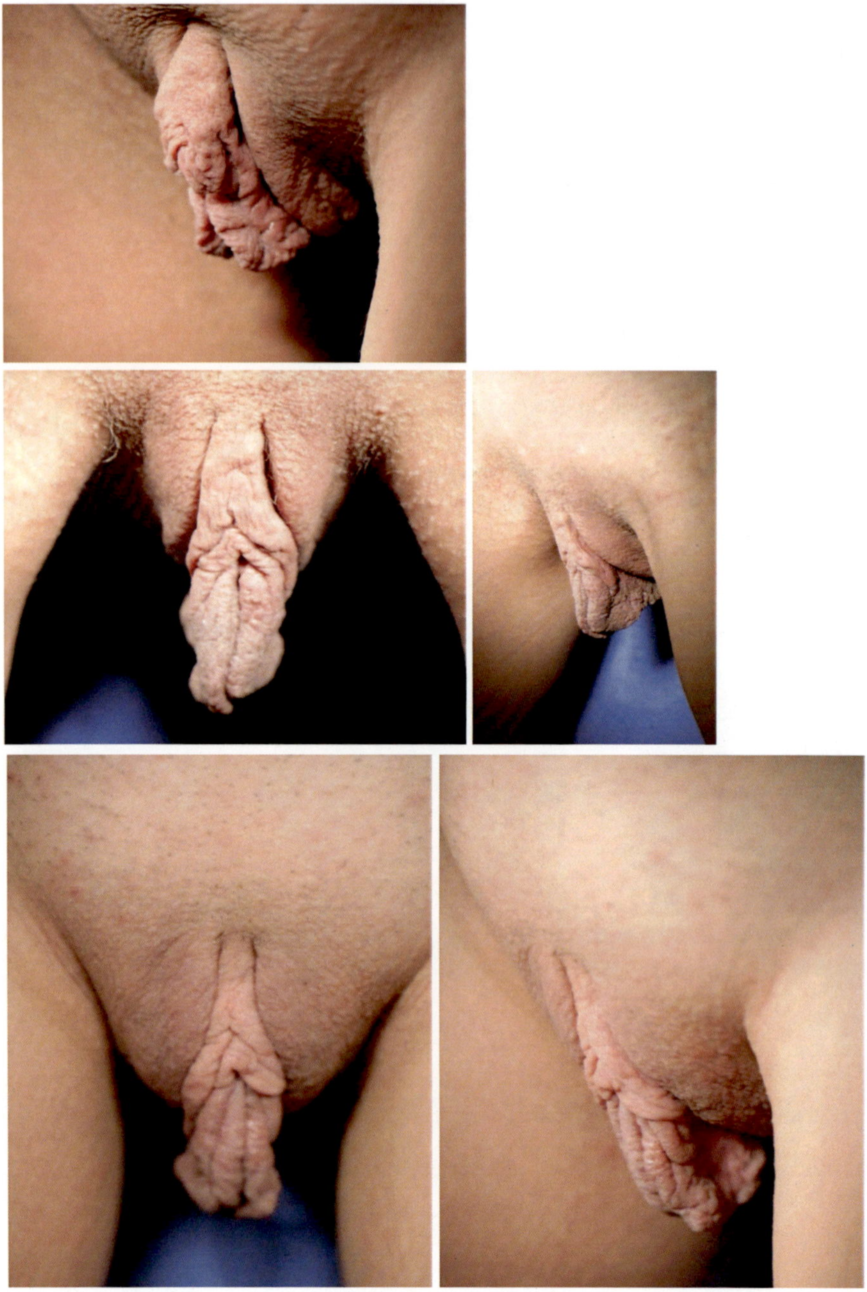

Fig. 12 (continued)

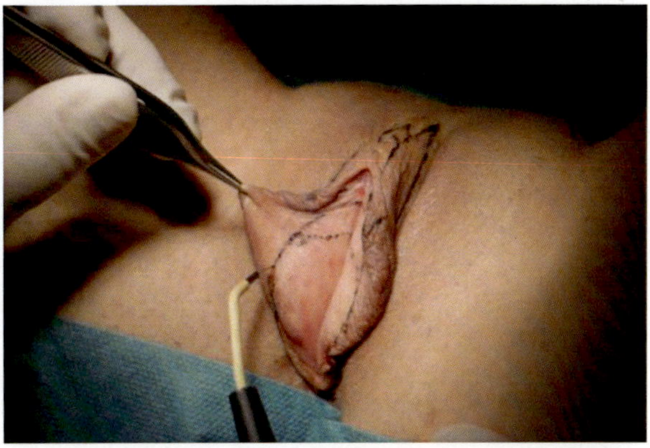

Fig. 13 Incision starting inferiorly

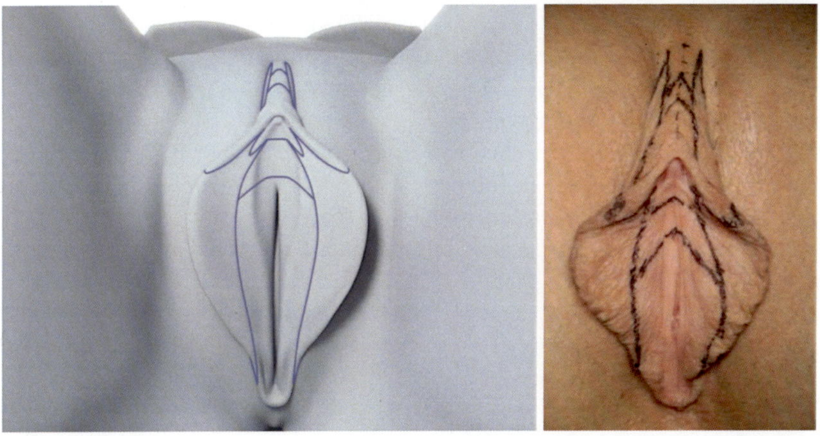

Fig. 14 Lines of skin incision, lithotomy position, frontal view

The labial height can be quite small towards the posterior commissure, about 2–3 mm. Severe postoperative tissue shrinkage is not to be expected here. The labial height increases progressively, reaching the required height just below the clitoris, and then decreases again slightly. In this way, the labia can be given a slight waviness. Shaping the labia minora is done mainly in this area. The maximum height of the labia is just below the clitoris and should ideally be about 8 mm to 10 mm, but may be more if the patient so wishes. This segment does shrink somewhat postoperatively, so take care not to overcorrect it.

The incision line on the inner aspect of the labium then encounters the tip of the frenulum of the clitoris. Cut around the frenulum on both sides in such a way as to form a sufficiently long triangular extension, which will later be inserted into the inner side of the labia. Cutting around the frenulum lateral to the glans can extend superiorly some 3–5 mm on the inner surface of the clitoral hood, but must be at least 2–3 mm from the lateral border of the glans, so as not to risk disrupting clitoral sensation. Medially the incision then runs below the glans, horizontally to the midline. Here, too, make sure there is a distance of at least 2–5 mm from the inferior border of the glans (Fig. 14).

Starting from the lateral line along the frenulum, the incision turns inferiorly to dissect out a flap measuring approximately 15 mm long and 6–7 mm wide, with its apex pointing downwards. This flap consists of the lateral aspect of the clitoral hood and of the upper part of the lower segment of the labia minora. It has a key role in tightening the labia. Make sure there is enough subcutaneous tissue beneath the skin of the flap, partly to prevent vascular compromise of the flap, as it will later be put under tension, and partly to have sufficient tissue available for the subcutaneous fixation of the flap (Fig. 15).

The incision is then directed superomedially towards the midline and runs vertically about 3–4 mm from the midline marking to reach the beginning of the interlabial fold at the top. The incision should not project beyond the interlabial fold as it would then be visible later.

The line of the incision then returns downwards, at first very briefly in the interlabial fold, and then medially along the clitoral shaft, slightly ascending to a height of about 3–4 mm from the level of the interlabial fold.

Half of the flap diameter is added to the definitive labial height at this point. In this segment, or just below the clitoris, the height of the labia minora measured from the interlabial fold is at its maximum.

To complete the incision, the outer aspect of the labium is incised in a slight curve corresponding to the line followed on the inner aspect, down to the level of the labia to be removed at the posterior end (Fig. 16).

To tighten the clitoral hood superiorly, a reflected rhomboid-shaped area is drawn in on the remaining strip of prepuce. The vertical measurement of this section corresponds roughly to the extent by which the clitoral hood will be lifted and

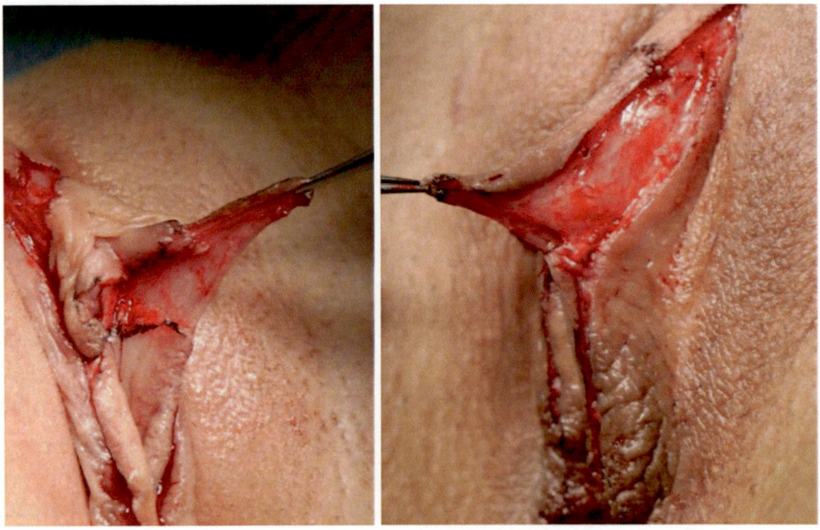

Fig. 15 Layer of subcutaneous tissue provides blood supply of the flap

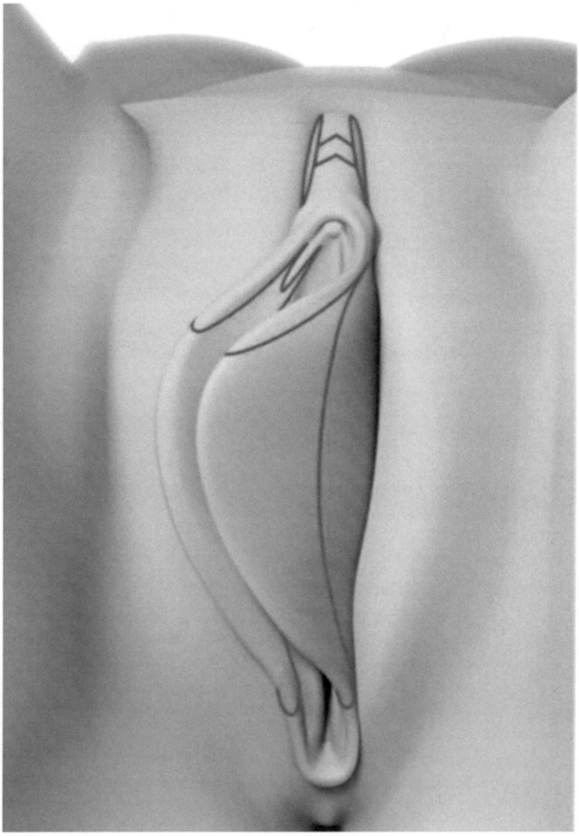

Fig. 16 Lines of incision

tightened. This section is pointed upwards in the midline, which will leave a triangular scar when the wound is closed. As with a rhinoplasty of the columella, a continuous horizontal scar across the prepuce should be avoided, as it may cause a very noticeable depression when the wound heals.

Any coagulation in the region of the clitoral shaft should be cautious and exclusively bipolar, so that there is no risk of clitoral sensation being disrupted by excessive coagulation (Figs. 17 and 24a).

For correction of clitoral protrusion, an arching line is drawn in to ascend medially from the marking on the inner aspect of each labium, following a path corresponding to that of the incision line medial to the frenulum just below the clitoris. The lines from the two sides meet in the midline and, together with the incision line below the clitoris, outline a trapezoidal area. The vertical measurement of this area gives the distance by which the clitoris will later be shifted downwards (Fig. 18).

When all areas are resected (Fig. 19a, b), three completely separate labial segments are created (Fig. 20a, b).

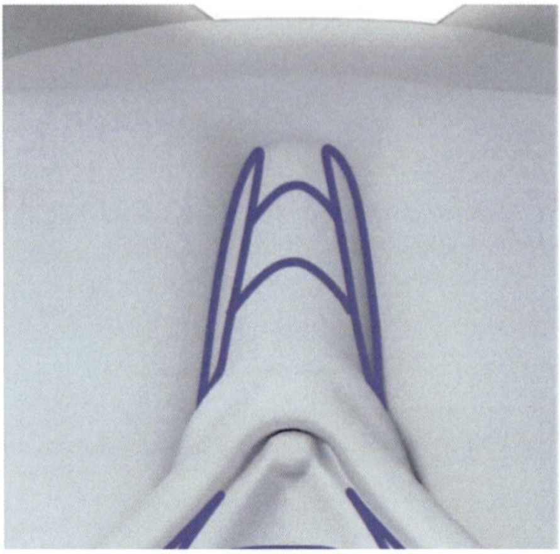

Fig. 17 Incision on the prepuce in shape of a reflected rhombus

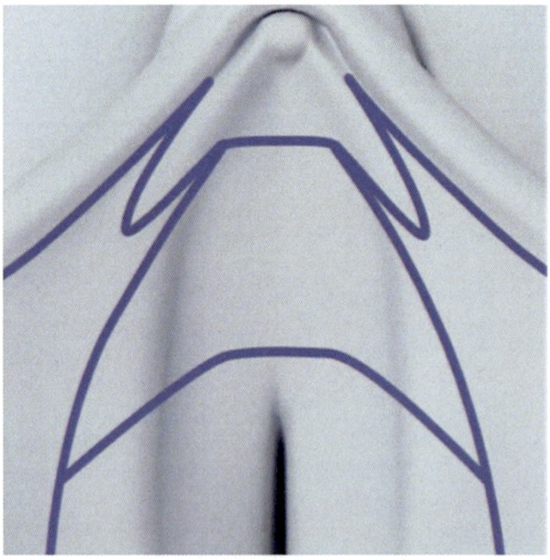

Fig. 18 Incisions following the frenulum and on the vaginal vestibule

Wound closure starts below the clitoris by suturing the subcutaneous tissue between the inner and outer aspects of the labium. We recommend a continuous suture technique with a 5–0 absorbable multifilament thread. This will catch most of the afferent blood vessels running perpendicularly in this area and reliably prevent postoperative bleeding (Fig. 21).

Then the segment around the prepuce is closed. One subcutaneous suture in the middle is usually sufficient to approximate the segment and take the tension off the skin. Close the skin from medial to lateral with 4–6 interrupted sutures using 6–0 absorbable monofilament thread (Fig. 22).

The tip (glans) of the clitoris is then shifted downwards. This is done by closing the segment below the clitoris (Fig. 23a, b) and (25a, b).

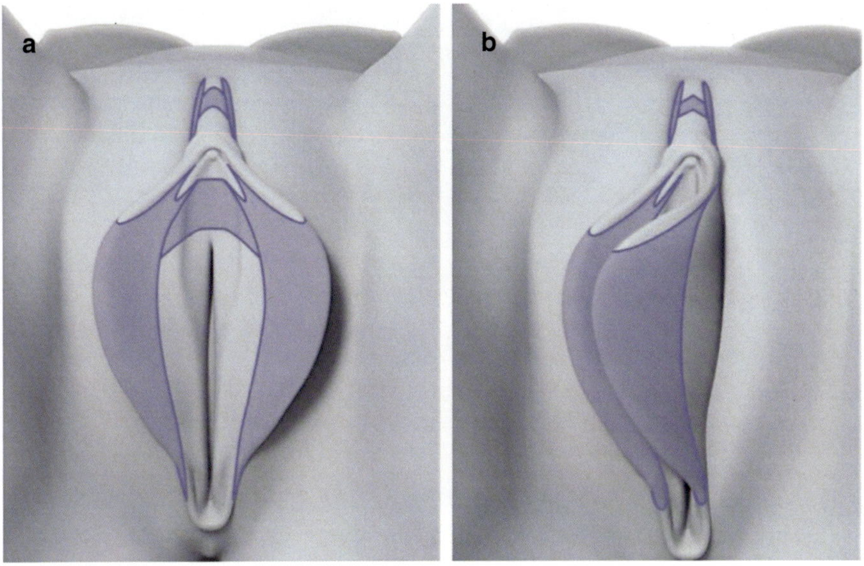

Fig. 19 (**a**) Area marked in dark blue is resected, frontal view, (**b**) Area marked in dark blue is resected, oblique view

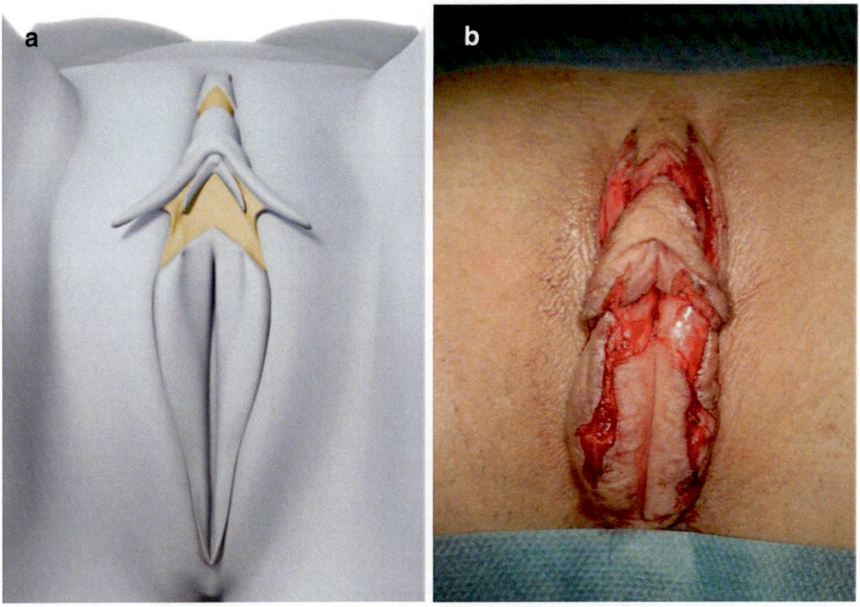

Fig. 20 (**a**) Three separate labial segments, frontal view (**b**) Intra operative view

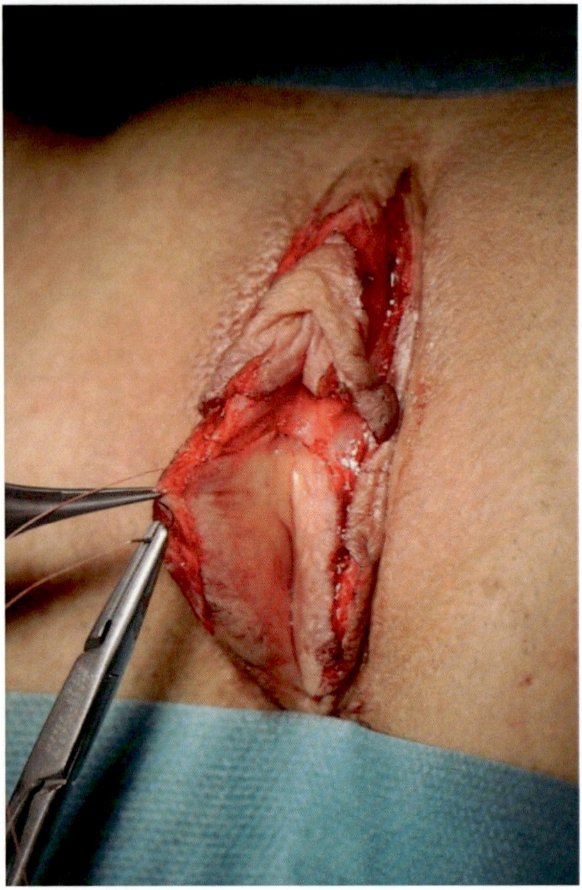

Fig. 21 Subcutaneous wound closure

Close the wound margins with interrupted sutures using a 4–0 or 5–0 multifilament thread. Place the middle suture first, preferably a mattress suture to provide the greatest possible stability. This central suture must be placed precisely in the midline, i.e. exactly beneath the middle of the glans clitoris and in line with the middle of the external urethral orifice; otherwise the clitoris may lie in an oblique position and cause the urine stream to deviate.

The skin resection should not reach closer than 1 cm above the external urethral orifice, as tension on the sutures could then affect the morphology and dynamics of the urinary meatus, likewise having irreversible effects on the direction of the urine stream.

As the closure of this segment is done under slight tension, it is advisable to place the sutures close together, to prevent postoperative wound dehiscence (Fig. 24).

The lateral flaps are now integrated into the line of the labia below the clitoris, between the outer and inner aspects of the labia minora. This part of the procedure is done under slight tension in order to achieve further tightening of the clitoral hood in a downward direction, in addition to the previous tightening directed upwards (Fig. 25a–e).

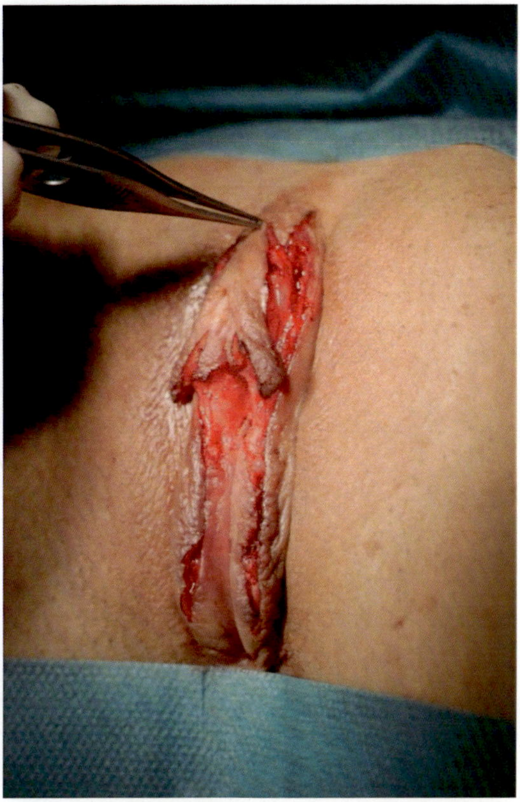

Fig. 22 Closing the preputial segment tightens the clitoral hood in an anterior direction

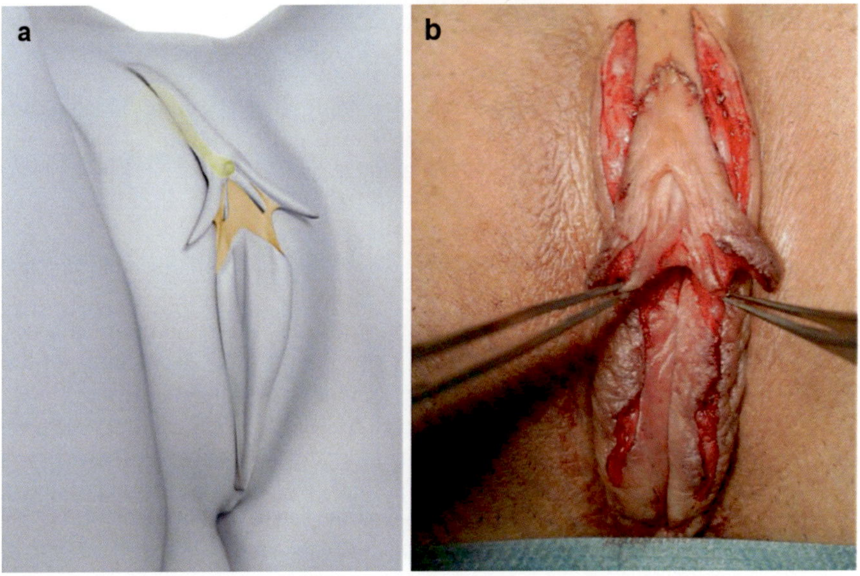

Fig. 23 (**a**, **b**) Closure of the segment below the clitoris shifts the glans in a posterior direction and corrects clitoral protrusion

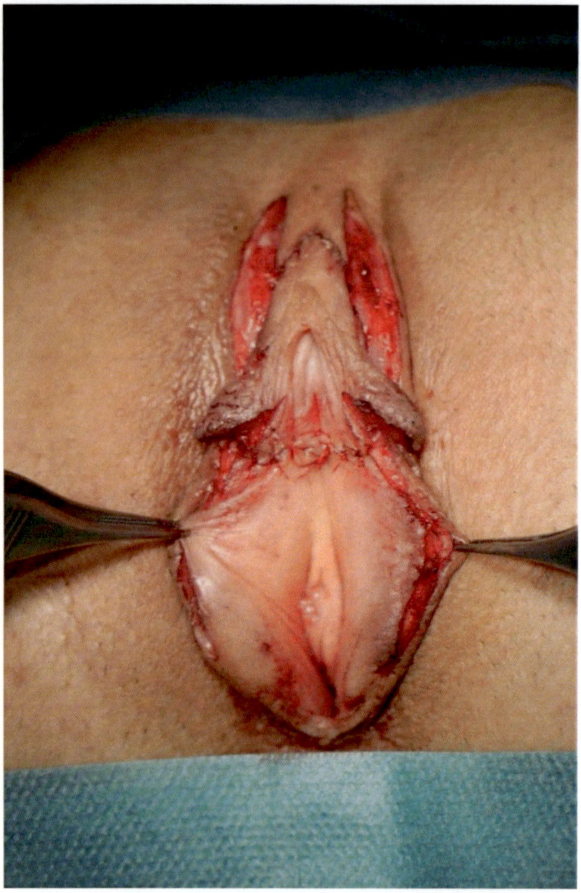

Fig. 24 Closure of the infra-clitoral segment

The tip of the flap is anchored with a 5–0 multifilament suture which can be interweaved with the previous subcutaneous labial suture, affording good stability for the fixation. Tensioning of the flap reduces the labial height somewhat, a factor that has to be taken into account in the preoperative planning and decision on the final labial height.

Dissection scissors can be used on both sides of the flap to mobilise the skin and, if necessary, to shorten it further. An excess of the skin can also be used to achieve a greater labial height and greater roundness of the labia in this region (Fig. 26a–d).

At this juncture, there is a possibility of shifting the level of the clitoral shaft somewhat downwards (inwards) within the sagittal plane (some downward movement of the clitoral shaft was already achieved by correcting the clitoral protrusion and by shortening the prepuce).

This is indicated particularly if the clitoral shaft protrudes, and it is impossible to achieve a narrow pudendal cleft by reducing the inner labia alone.

Use dissection scissors to spread the subcutaneous tissue parallel to the clitoral shaft, and create an opening on the dorsal aspect of the lateral crus or on the lateral aspects of the clitoral body. Use a 4–0 or 5–0 absorbable multifilament suture to

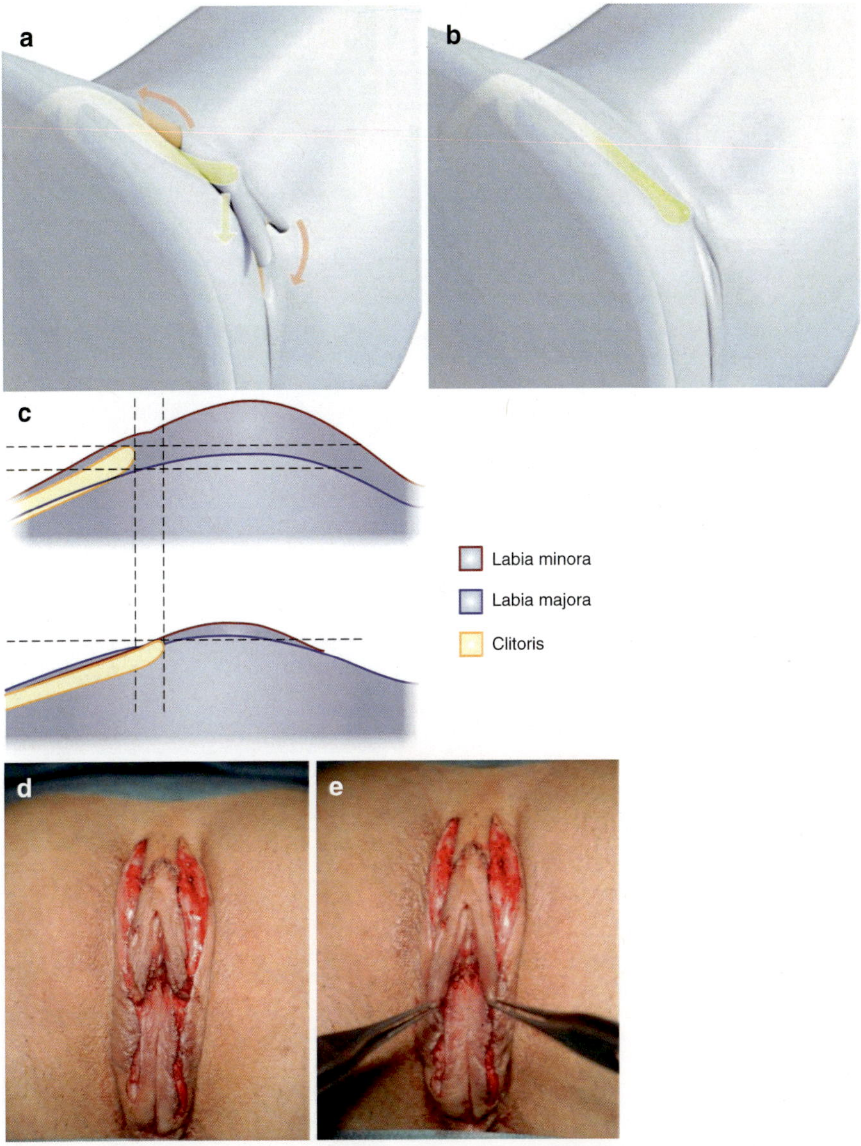

Fig. 25 (**a**) Tightening the clitoral hood by superior and inferior tension (*orange arrows*) and shifting the glans of the clitoris downwards in a sagittal and frontal plane (*yellow arrow*) corrects clitoral protrusion and clitoral hood hypertrophy. (**b**) More inferior position of the glans of the clitoris. (**c**) Lateral view: reduction of the labia minora with shifting the clitoris downwards in a sagittal plane. Clitoris (*yellow*). Labia minora (*red*), Labia majora (*blue*). (**d**) Downward directed tension on the lateral flaps allows additional tightening of the clitoral hood. (**e**) Inserted lateral flaps

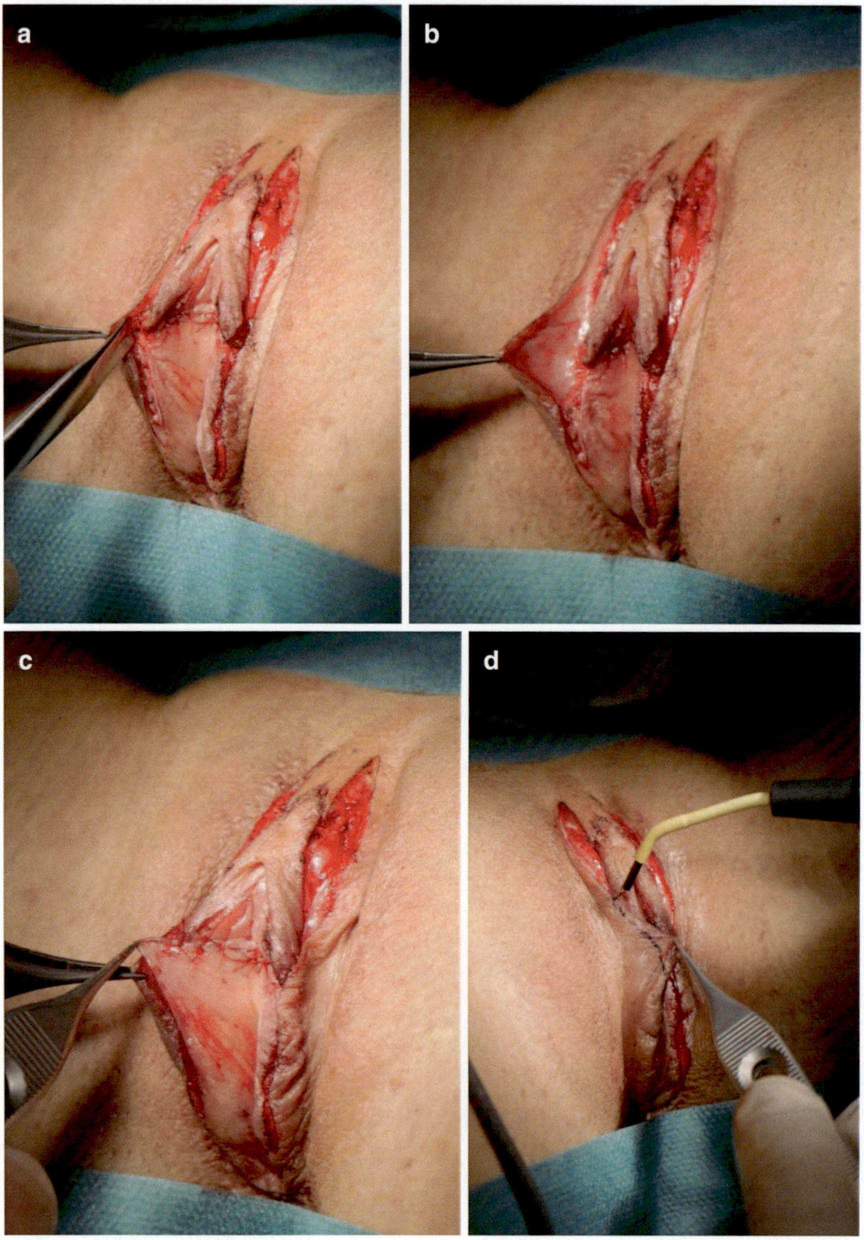

Fig. 26 (**a**–**d**) Release of the skin medially and laterally to the flap with trimming and contour shaping (oblique view right)

grasp the tunica albuginea of the crus or body of the clitoris and then the lateral and medial edges of the wound above and distal to the fusion line on the clitoral shaft. By pulling on the knot, the clitoral shaft will migrate a few millimetres downwards in the sagittal plane (inwards) (Fig. 27a–f).

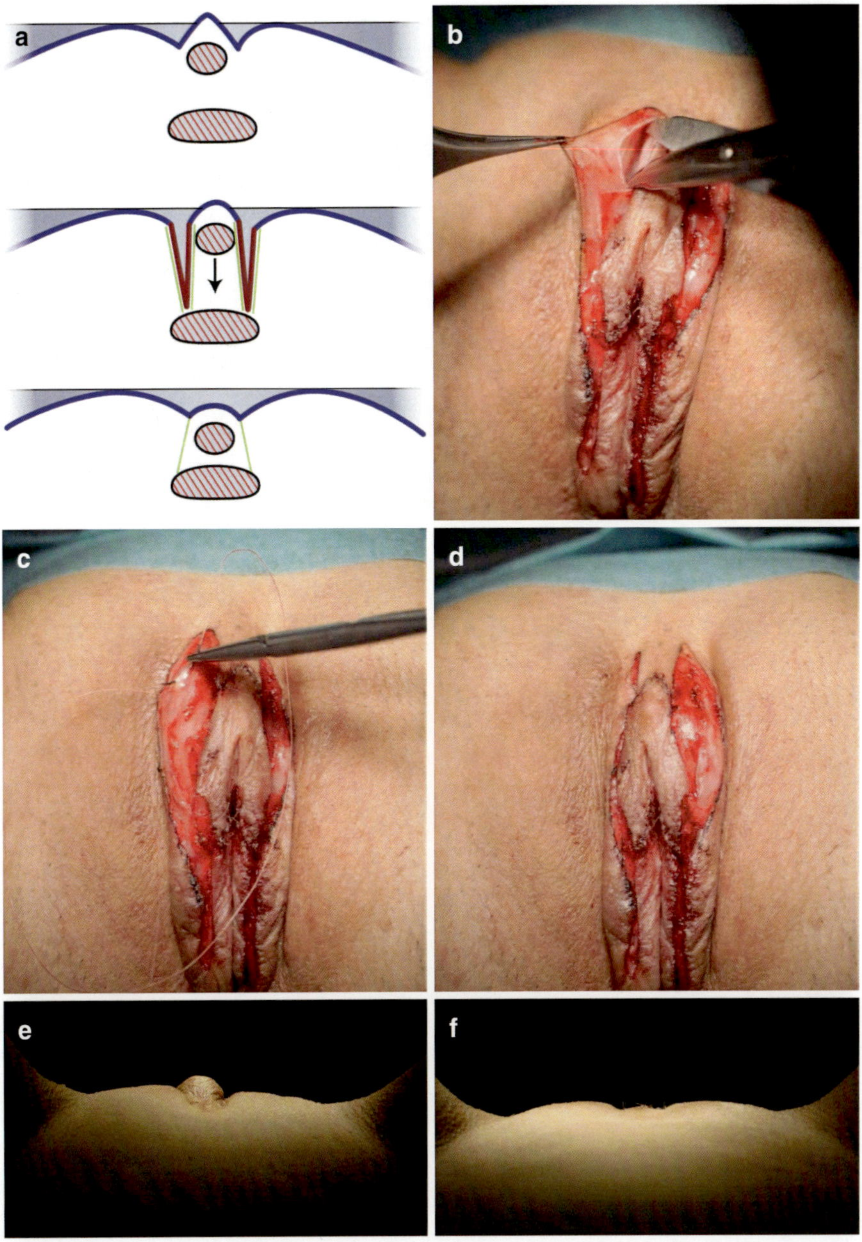

Fig. 27 (**a**) Tightening stitches placed into the tunica albuginea of the crura or the clitoral body pulls the clitoral shaft inwards. (**b**) Use spreading scissor action for the preparation of the clitoral body or crus (**c**) Placing a suture into the tunica albuginea and into the wound edges. (**d**) Closing the knot pulls the clitoral shaft inwards (here on the right side). (**e**) Protruding clitoral shaft from cranial view before surgery. (**f**) Clitoral shaft after surgery, same view

Now start the skin closure on the inner aspect of the flap. Close the skin as precisely as possible with a continuous suture using a fine 6–0 monofilament thread, so that the lateral flap heals without creating a step in the smooth line of the labia.

A continuous (running) suture is the best technique to use for almost all skin closures, as it is relatively stable and can withstand the mechanical forces due to movement that always affect the genital area during the postoperative healing phase. Nevertheless, the spaces between the needle entry points may swell (giving the appearance of a string of pearls). As a rule, these swellings usually disappear completely. Even though a simple closely spaced running stitch is generally the suture of choice, a continuous mattress suture is the better technique to use in the labial segment below the clitoris, i.e. along the free edge, as this reduces the risk of unsightly uneven contours and reliably produces a smooth wound edge. A 6–0 absorbable monofilament suture is the most suitable for this purpose.

After closing the skin, start below the clitoris and place mattress sutures close together through the inner and outer aspects of the labium, to shape, lift, and stabilise the labial walls. Continue as far as the posterior commissure. The knots should lie on the inner aspect of the labium. Use 5–0 absorbable multifilament sutures.

This last and extremely important step gives additional shape to the labia minora, prevents them being pulling apart and flattened by swelling, and helps them to heal in an erect position (Fig. 28a–c).

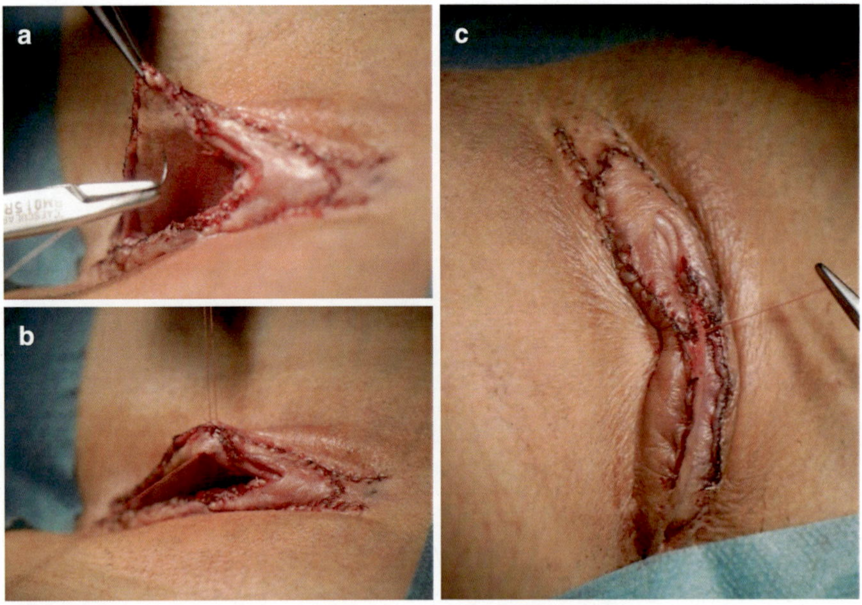

Fig. 28 Mattress sutures. (**a**) Passing the needle through the inner aspect first. (**b**) Inserted mattress suture. (**c**) Tightening the knot erects and stabilizes the labial wall. images directly before and after surgery, lithotomy position. Frontal view, Oblique view left

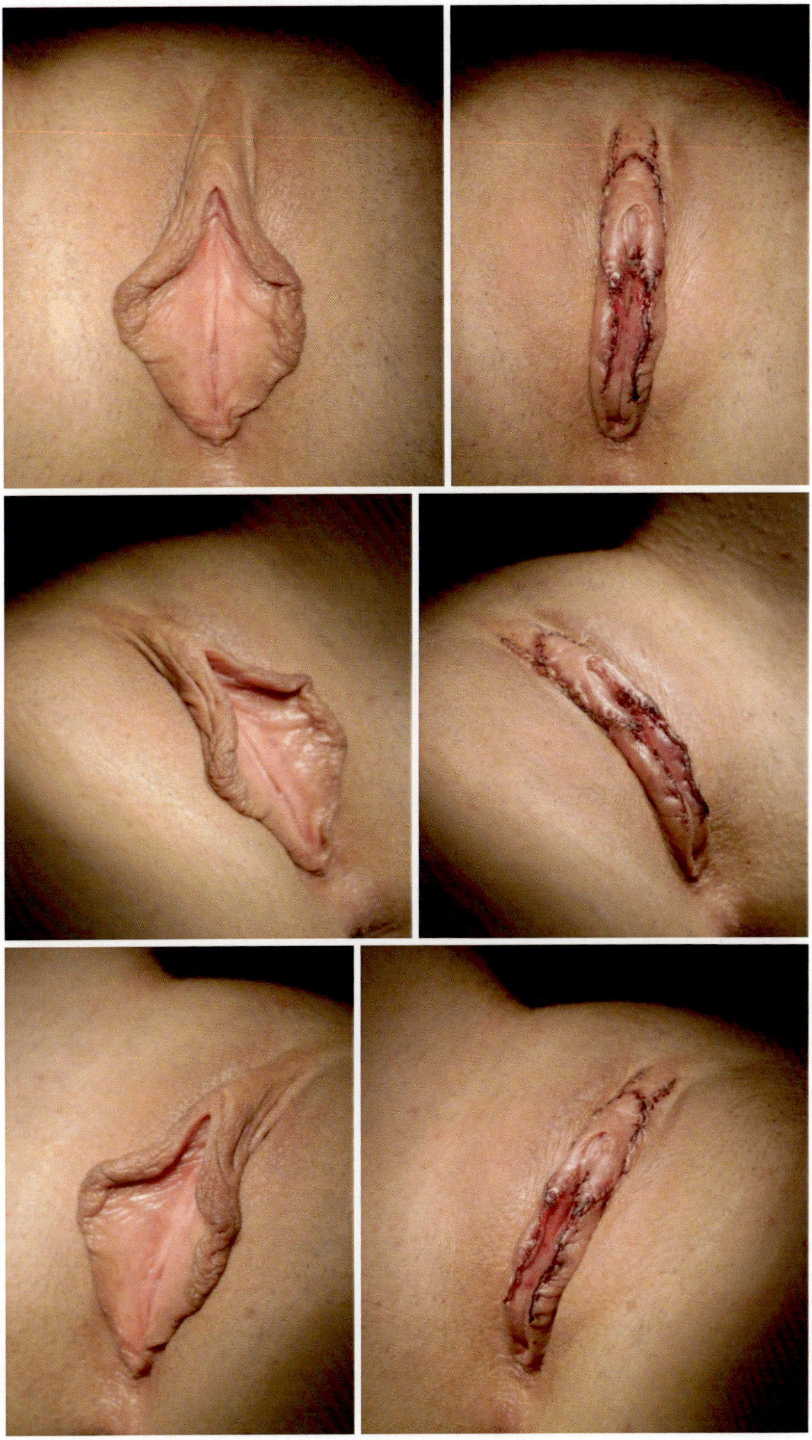

Fig. 28 (continued)

Examples results composite reduction labiaplasty CRL
Patient 1
Pre-OP Standing

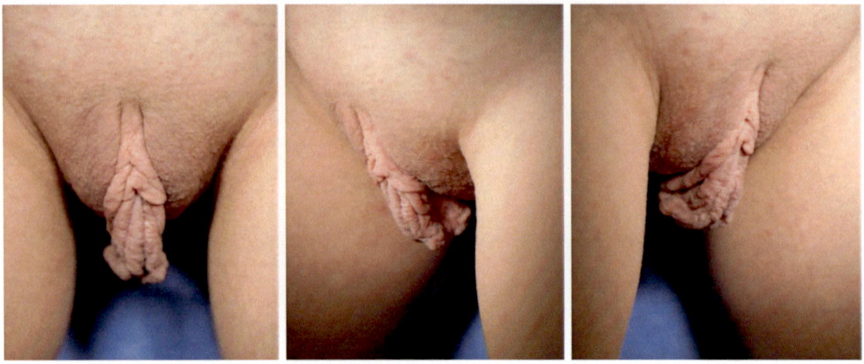

Pre-OP Lithotomy-Position

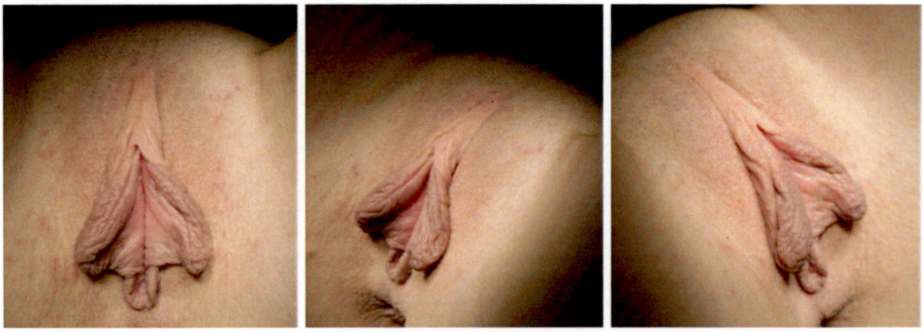

Immediate Post-OP lithotomy position

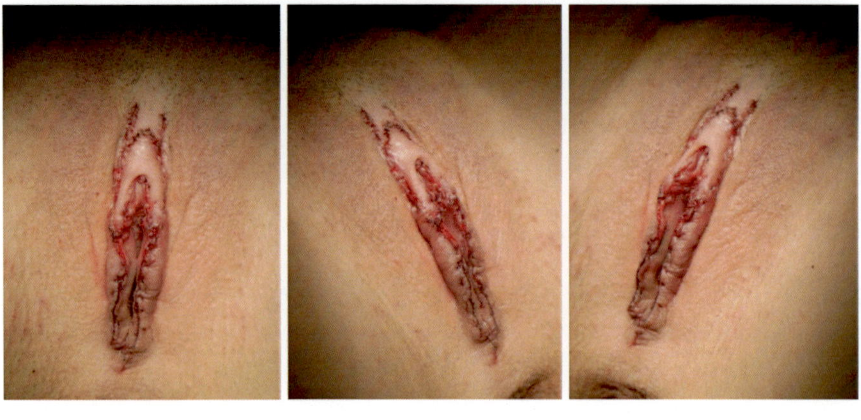

Long term post OP standing

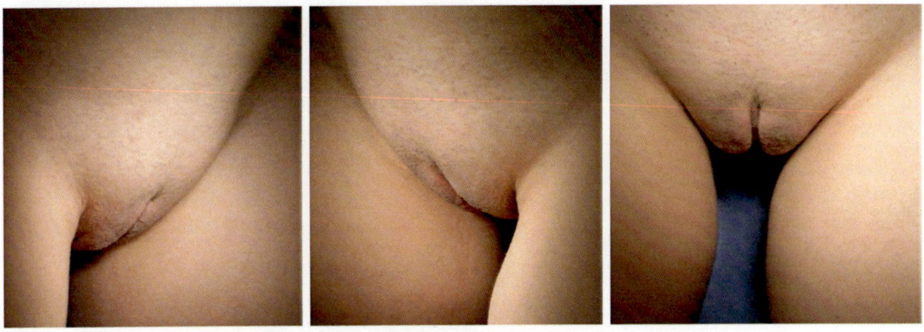

Long term post-OP lithotomy position

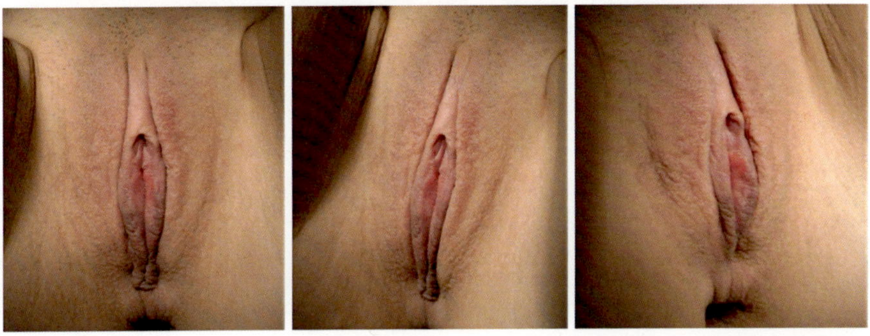

Patient 2

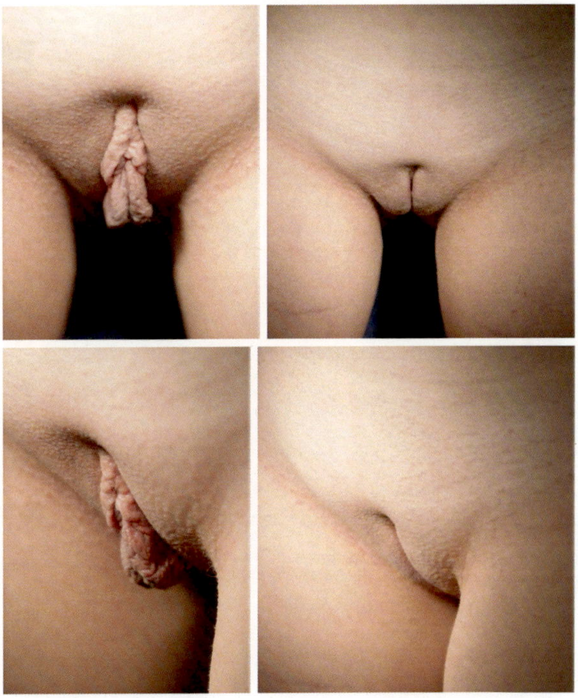

Patient 3

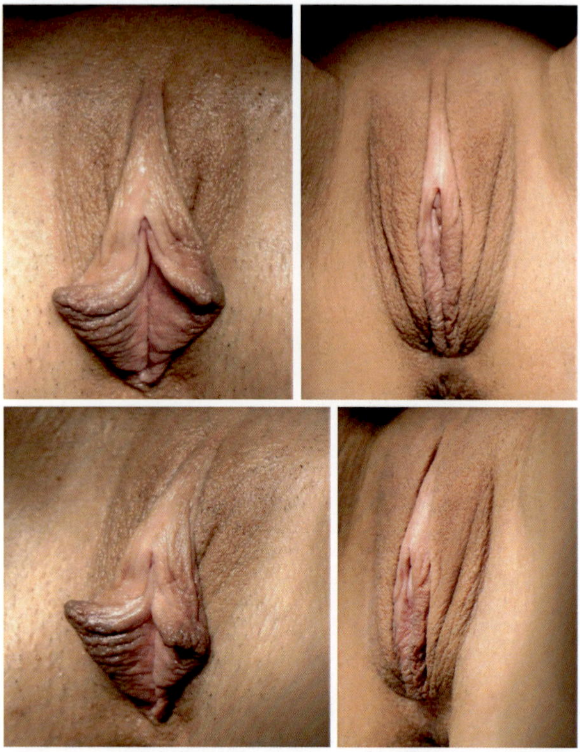

Patient 4

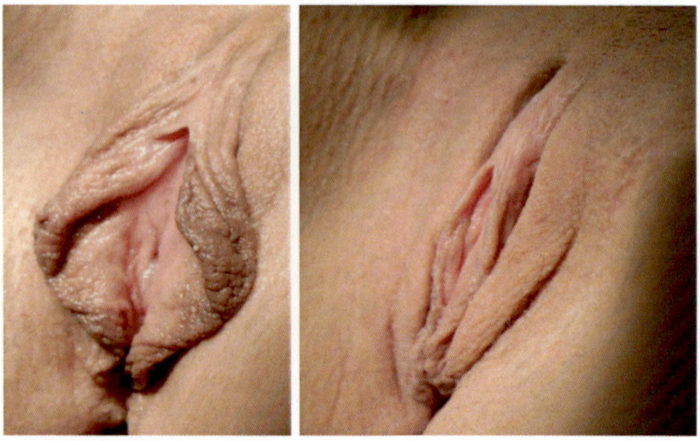

Labia Minora Reduction along the Entire Length with Correction of the Position of the Clitoris

Indication

This technique is similar to the *composite reduction labiaplasty* but with the difference that there is no additional upward tightening of the clitoral hood. The patient should not have an overhanging clitoral hood in need of correction and a short clitoral shaft with a short or normal length of prepuce. This method is indicated for hypertrophy of the labia minora in all three segments, i.e. above and below the clitoris as well as at the level of the clitoris and in cases of clitoral protrusion (Fig. 29).

Operation

Resection also starts at the posterior commissure and follows a slightly curving path towards the frenulum of the clitoris. Once again, the frenulum is dissected out into a long inferior extension, and a lateral flap consisting of the distal extension of the clitoral hood is also fashioned on each side.

The incision then runs up towards the anterior commissure parallel to the midline of the clitoral shaft and, at the origin of the interlabial fold, turns back inferiorly in it, then ascending again to meet the resection line on the outer aspect of the labium, a little below the clitoris.

To shift the level of the tip of the clitoris downwards, a trapezoidal section of the skin is removed from below the clitoris; the width of this section determines the distance by which the tip of the clitoris will migrate downwards (Fig. 30).

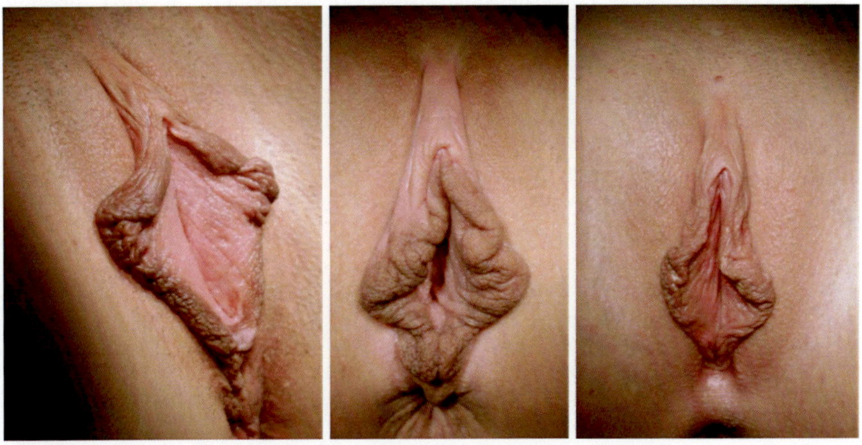

Fig. 29 Patients with hypertrophy of the labia minora in all segments, clitoral protrusion, short or normal length prepuce, no descending clitoral hood

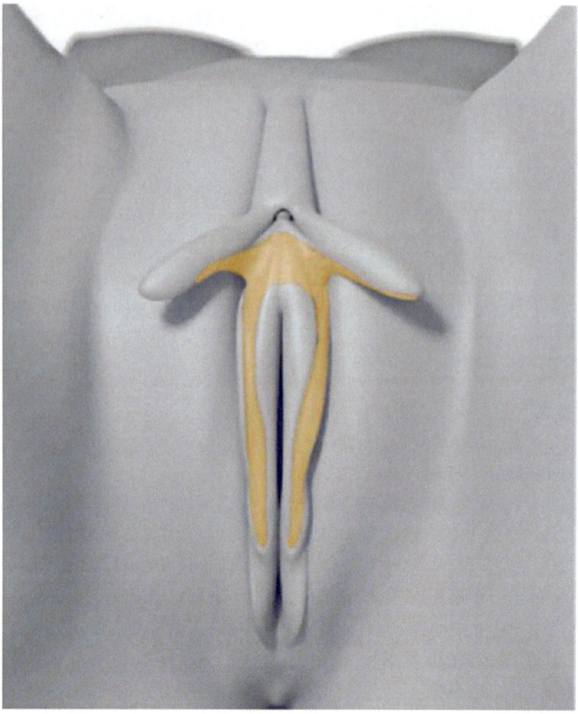

Fig. 30 The width of the skin resected at the viganal vestibule determines the downward migration of the clitoris (descending part and glans)

The lateral flaps are then integrated into the line of the labia and fixed subcutaneously with 5–0 absorbable multifilament sutures under moderate tension.

After mobilising the inner and outer aspects of the labia in this area, the labial height and shape below the clitoris can be manipulated very well at this juncture.

After closing the wound as described previously, the final step is also to hold the labial wall erect with closely placed through-and-through mattress sutures using 5–0 absorbable multifilament thread.

Examples
Patient 1

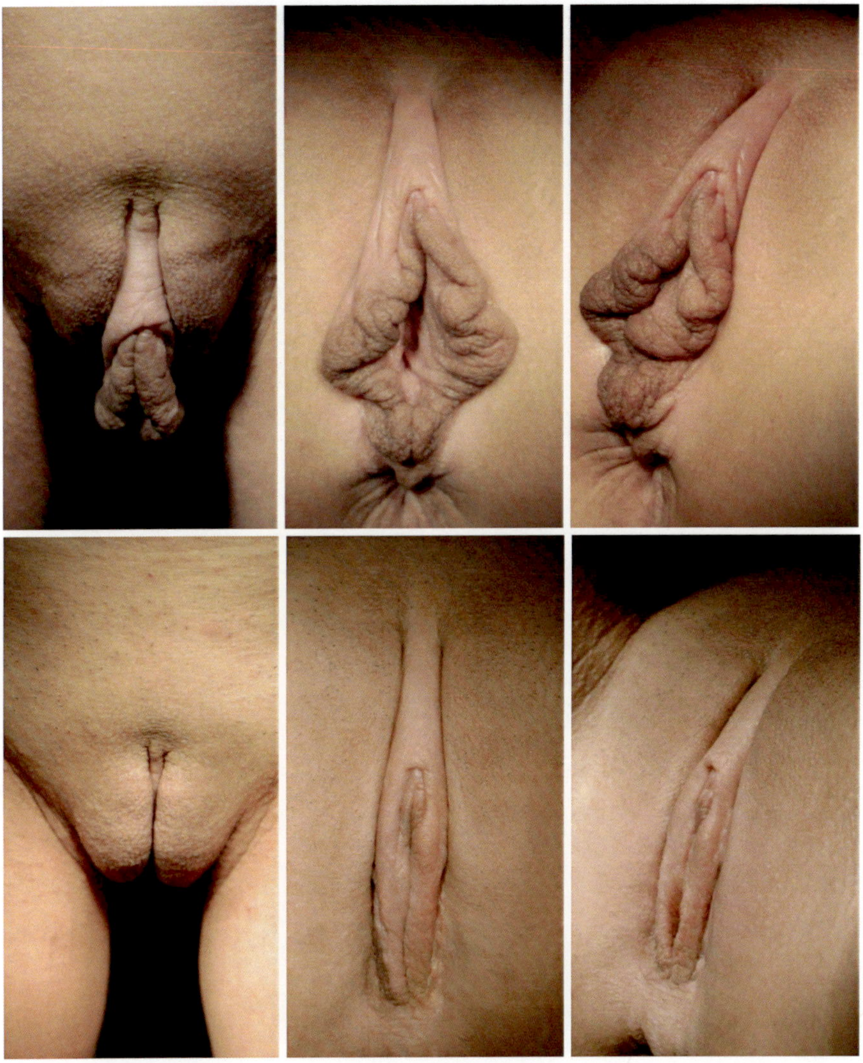

Examples
Patient 2

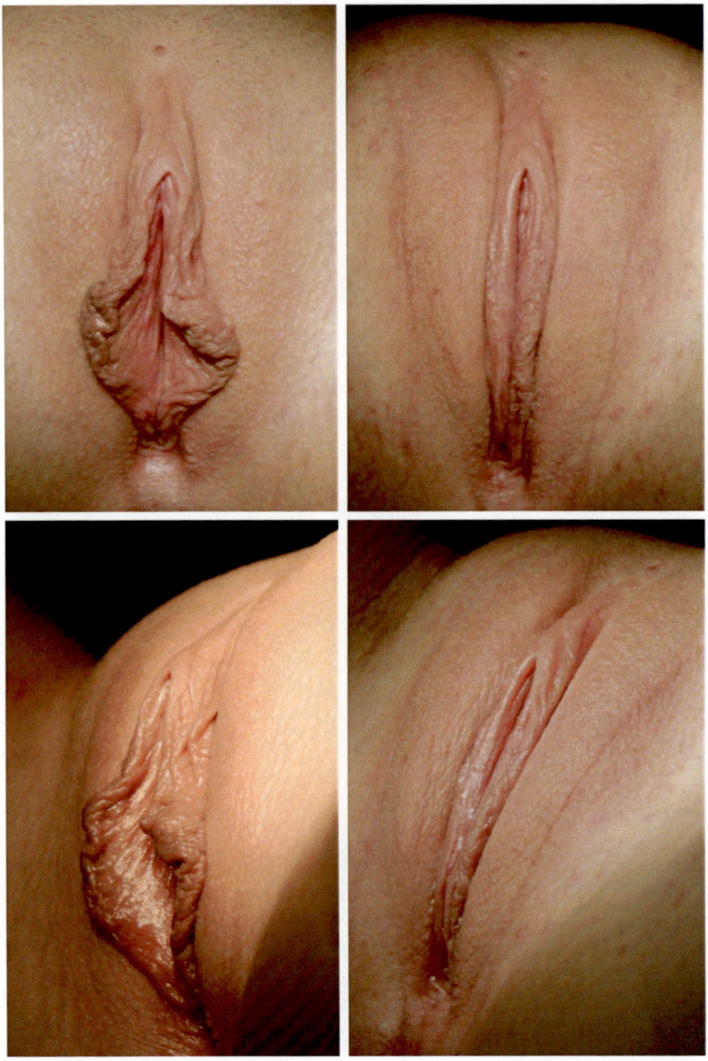

Examples
Patient 3

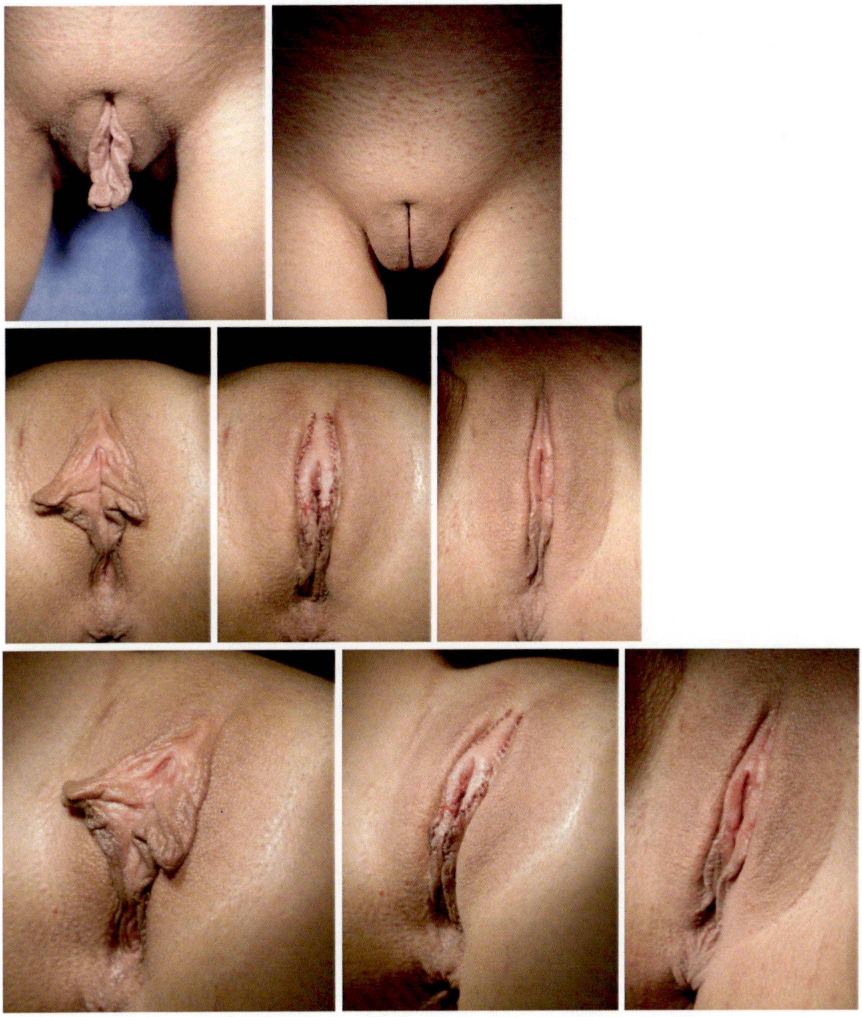

Labia Minora Reduction along the Entire Length without Correction of the Position of the Clitoris

Indication

This is the method of choice when there is hypertrophy of the labia minora in all segments but no other concerns. There is no overhanging clitoral hood in need of tightening, no long preputial segment due to a long clitoral shaft, and no clitoris protrusion that has to be corrected (Fig. 31).

Operation

After marking the lines, the incision starts in the lower labial segment and, like the other variants, runs superiorly towards the frenulum in a slight curve. However, in this case, the frenulum is not dissected out into a long triangle. Instead, the incision continues along the frenulum and, shortly before reaching the glans clitoris, turns steeply downwards at a sharp angle directed slightly laterally, to form the lateral flap as described previously. By removing the tissues between these lines, the frenulum is slightly reduced in height.

After cutting around the lateral flap, the incision continues upwards, lateral to the clitoral shaft, as far as the origin of the inner labium, where it then turns distally in the interlabial fold, ascending slightly in order to meet the incision line on the outer aspect of the labium minora a little below the level of the clitoris.

As the tension exerted on the lateral flap when it is integrated into the labium causes some tissue congestion, a Burow triangle with its apex pointing medially is excised from the inner aspect of the labium, about 1 cm below the clitoris (Fig. 32a–c).

This method also requires interrupted mattress sutures with 5–0 absorbable thread placed at close intervals to stabilise the labial wall and hold it erect.

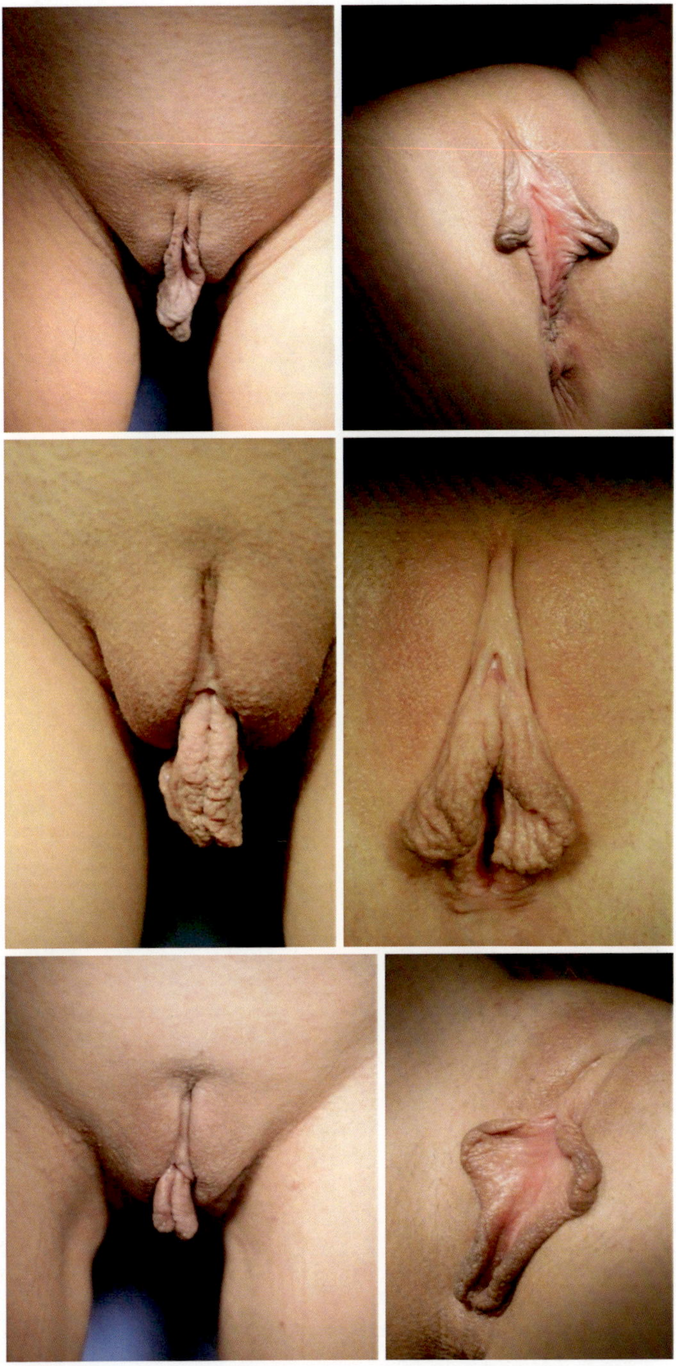

Fig. 31 Patients with labia hypertrophy in all segments, no descending clitoral hood, normal or short length prepuce, no clitoral protrusion

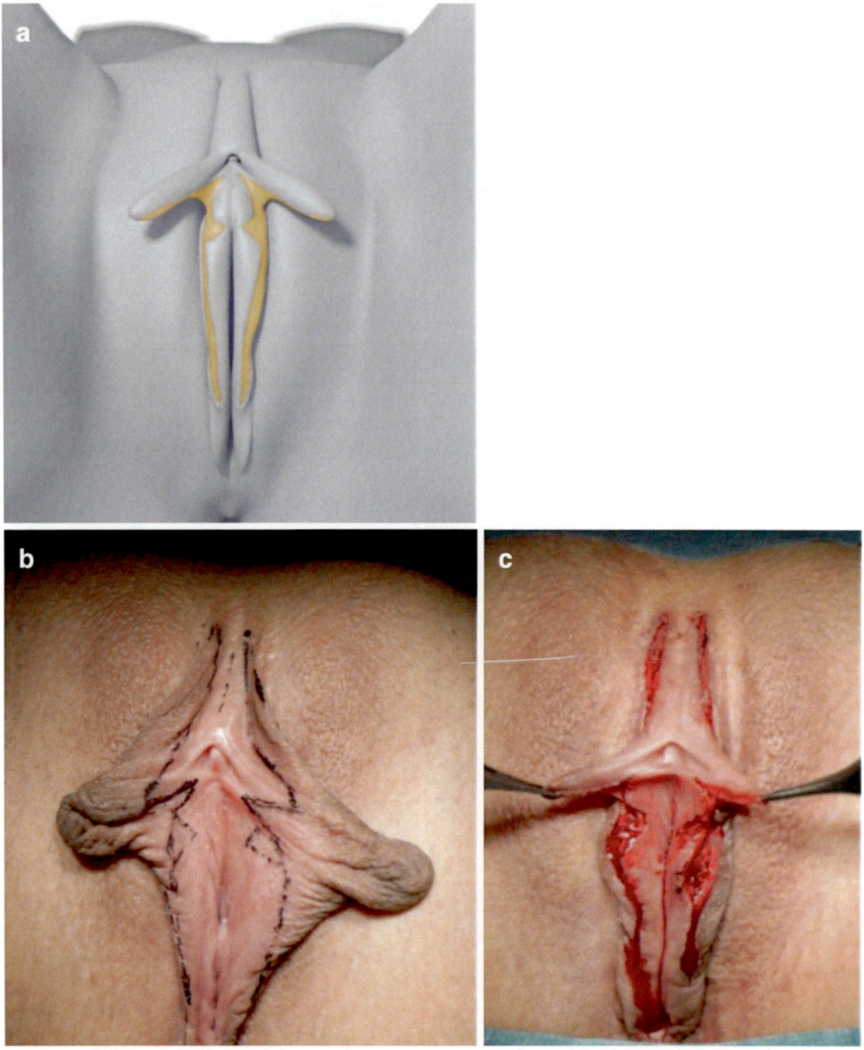

Fig. 32 (**a**–**c**) Removal of *Burow triangles* from the inner aspect of the labium

Examples
Patient 1

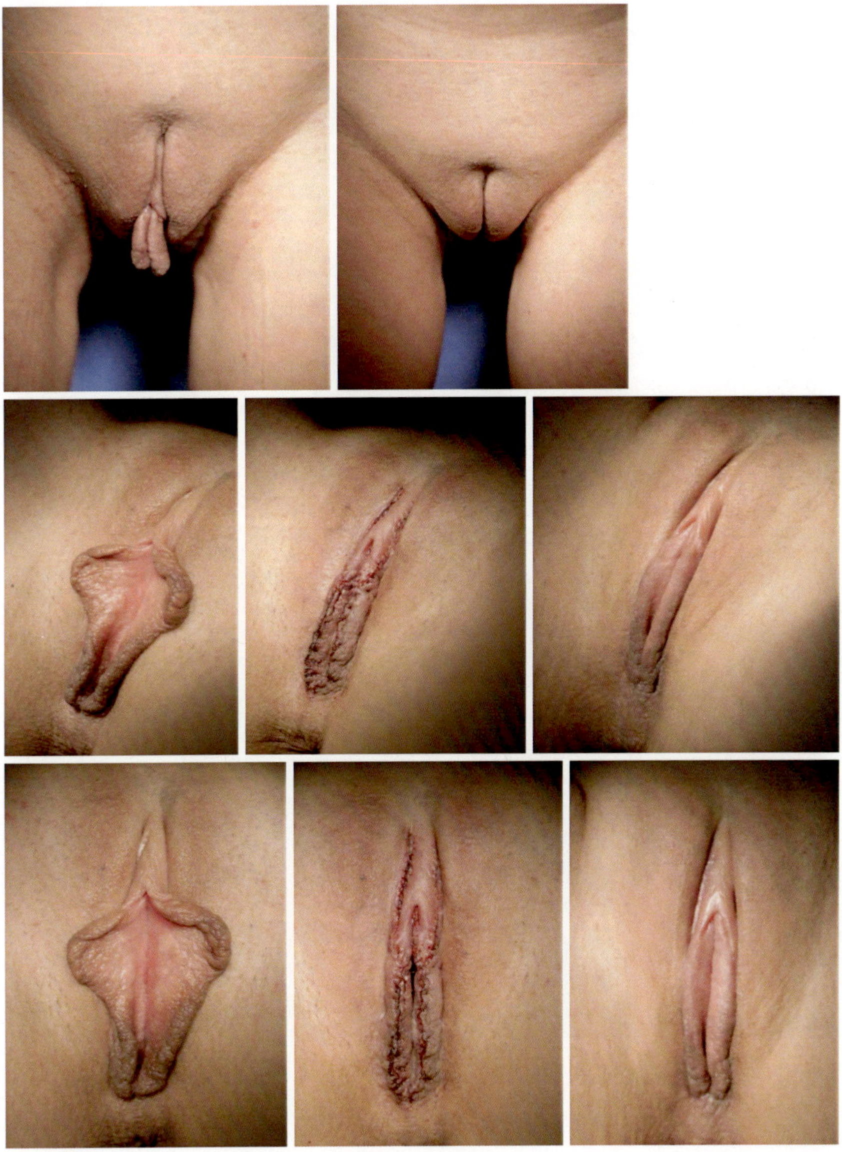

Examples
Patient 2

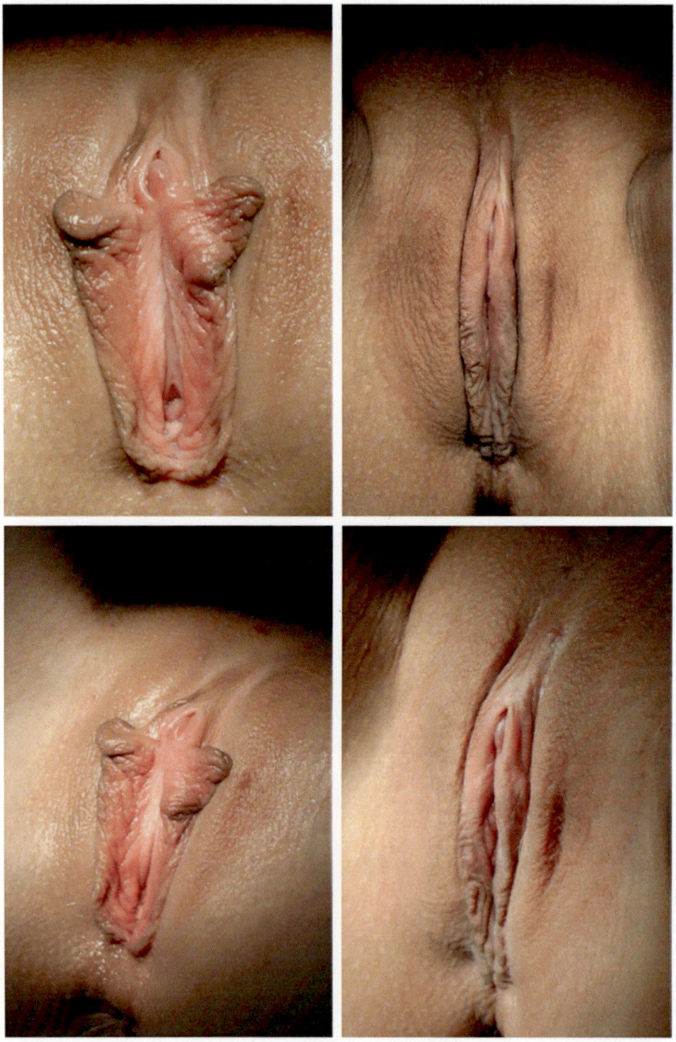

Labia Minora Reduction Only Distal to the Clitoris

Indication

As isolated hypertrophy of the labia minora distal to the clitoris is very rare, this variant is not frequently used.

It is the method of choice for hypertrophy confined to the distal segment, i.e. affecting the labia only below the level of the clitoris, without any clitoral protrusion or hyperplasia of the prepuce and the clitoral hood (Fig. 33).

Operation

Once again, the incision begins at the distal end of the labia and runs superiorly towards the frenulum describing a slight curve. On reaching the frenulum, however, the incision turns back and runs no further towards the base of the glans, as in the variant described above. The incision then turns distally, creating a lateral flap from the labial wall, although it is considerably shorter than the ones fashioned in the techniques described previously. This lateral flap is not inserted under tension, as there is no need to tighten the clitoral hood (Fig. 34a, b).

After creating the small flap, the incision again runs slightly superiorly but this time turns back inferiorly a little above the level of the glans clitoris to meet the incision line started in the distal segment on the outer aspect of the labium (Fig. 35).

Stabilising absorbable mattress sutures are also required along the base of the labia.

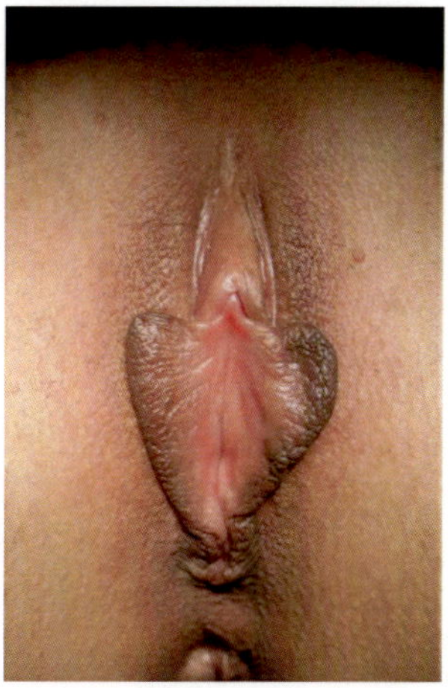

Fig. 33 Isolated hypertrophy in the segment below the clitoris, no clitoral protrusion, normal or short length prepuce

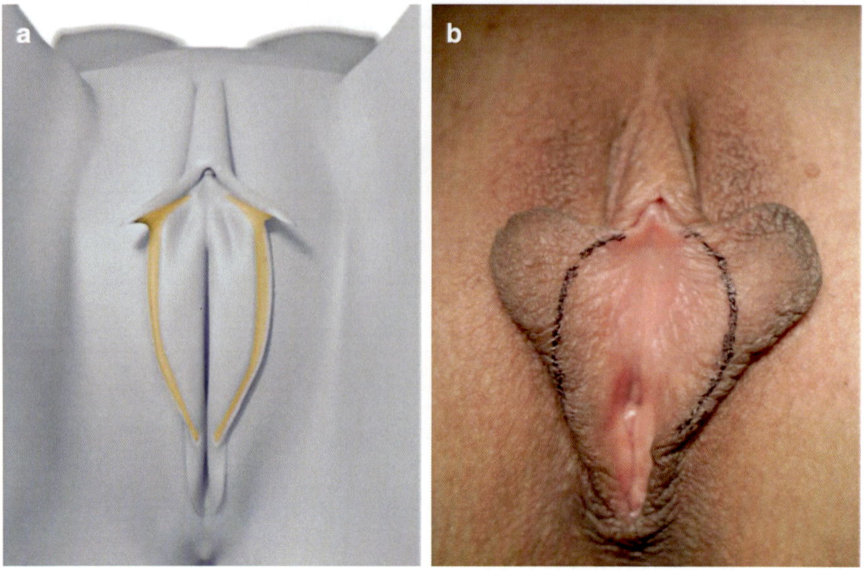

Fig. 34 (**a**, **b**) Resection of the labia minora only inferior to the clitoris creating two small lateral flaps, frontal view

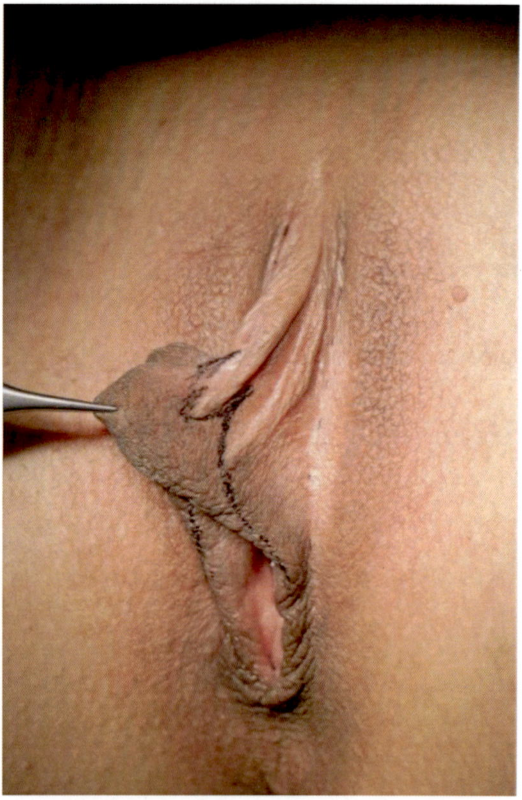

Fig. 35 Lateral view showing the incision line. The lateral flap is smaller compared to the techniques described above

Example

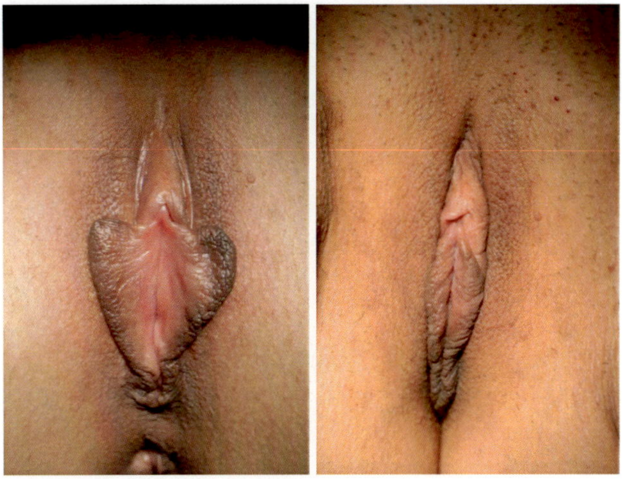

Labial Hypertrophy in the Region of the Posterior Commissure

Indication

One variation of normal, which is not infrequently seen, is hyperplasia of the labia minora in the region of the posterior commissure. The excess labial tissue often extends along the raphe across the perineum as far as the anus.

This excess tissue should always be corrected, as aesthetically it can be very unsightly, especially if this section is not treated when the rest of the labia are reshaped (Fig. 36).

To obtain an aesthetically pleasing result, excise a diamond-shaped section of tissue with the upper part of the diamond in the introitus and the lower part lying across the perineum (Fig. 37).

It is also possible to correct a dilated introitus or gaping vaginal vestibule, if the diamond shape is made correspondingly wide. Likewise, the bulbospongiosus muscle can be tightened medially during this procedure.

Operation

After marking the area, the skin is excised with the high-frequency unit. Depending on the tension required, use 3–0 or 4–0 absorbable sutures for the subcutaneous approximation of the wound margins. Close the wound with a continuous 6–0 absorbable monofilament suture to the skin (Fig. 38a, b).

Reinsertion of the labia minora into the posterior commissure should be directed somewhat medially and inferiorly, to prevent a bridge of the skin forming along the lower vaginal pole, which may be bothersome and painful during sexual intercourse (Fig. 39).

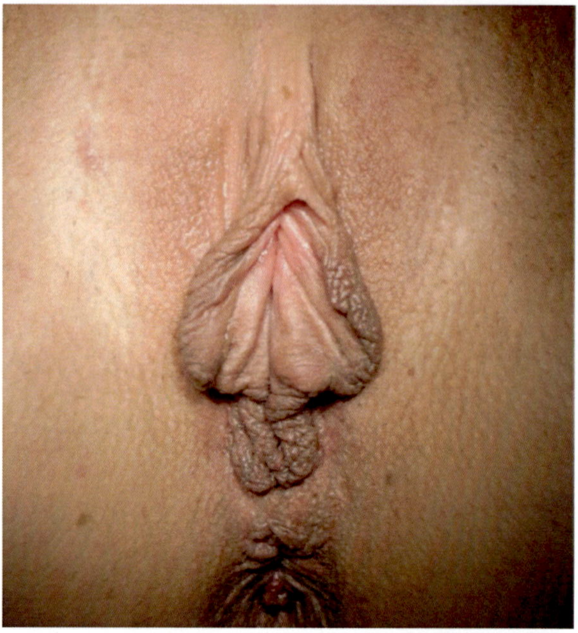

Fig. 36 Labia hypertrophy in the region of the posterior commissure

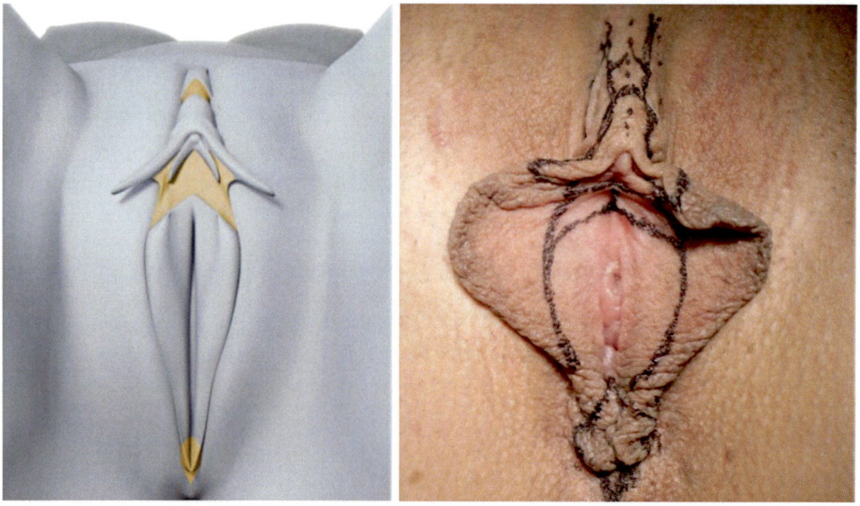

Fig. 37 Diamond-shaped excision in the posterior commissure (here in combination with *composite reduction labiaplasty*)

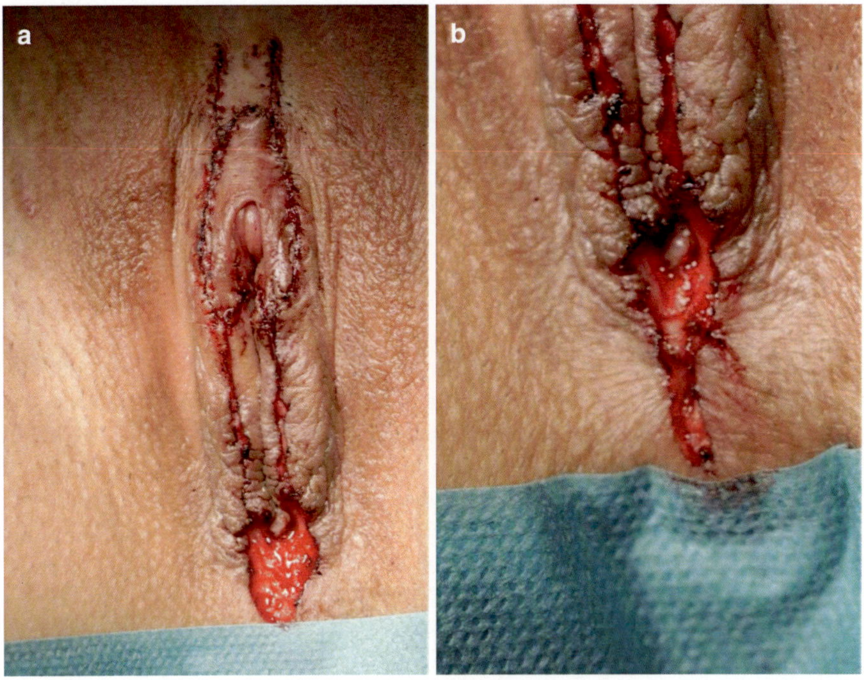

Fig. 38 (**a**) situation after labial excision at the posterior commissure. (**b**) approximation of wound edges

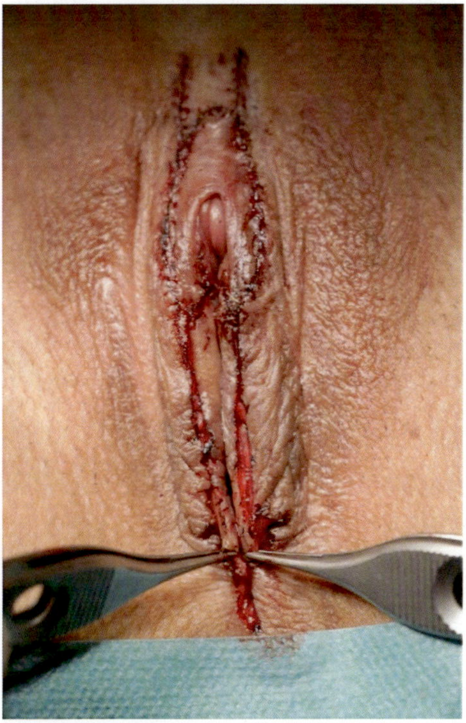

Fig. 39 Reinsertion of the posterior part of the labia minora under vertical tension

Dressings

Any blood residues should be cleaned from the area with hydrogen peroxide. Another injection of local anaesthetic ensures that there is no pain for a while.

Dressings consist of gauze compresses soaked with an alcohol-free mucosal disinfectant that has a cooling effect and reduces swelling in addition to disinfecting the wound. The gauze compresses are held in place with disposable mesh panties (hospital pants) (Fig. 40).

Postoperative Management

After the procedure, give the patient time to recover in the practice before she goes home or back to her hotel. Cool the genital area during this time. Before leaving the clinic, the patient should go to the toilet and then have a fresh dressing applied, so that she can keep this new dressing on for as long as possible. Wearing firm panties with even pressure over the genital area is recommended for the first night after surgery, in order to reduce the swelling as much as possible and minimise the chances of postoperative bleeding. Make sure that the patient has an adequate supply of analgesics, e.g. ibuprofen 600 and metamizole, as postoperative pain has always to be reckoned with.

Check the wound the following day, disinfect the area with a mucosal disinfectant, and apply a fresh dressing. The patient can then be discharged until the next follow-up visit.

Especially after a labia minora reduction, the patient should wear a gauze compress between the labia, to prevent them touching each other, for 14 days after

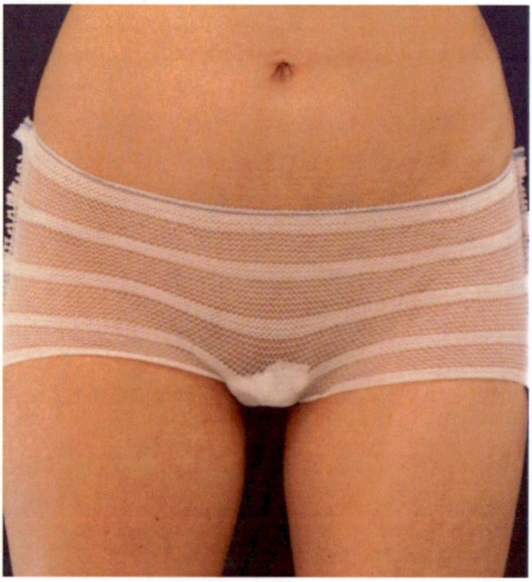

Fig. 40 Dressing

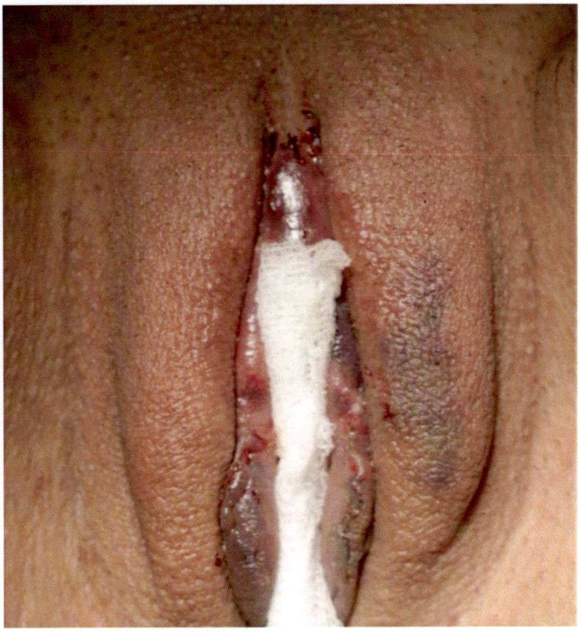

Fig. 41 Gauze held between the labia for stabilization and contouring

surgery. This prevents one labium slipping under the other, which would lead to the two sides healing differently and result in an asymmetry that would be hard or even impossible to correct with conservative treatment (Fig. 41).

After these first 2 weeks, the patient can apply pressure to the labia, to make the swelling go down quicker and provide optimal conditions for the wound to heal. Each side should be squeezed along its length between the index finger and the thumb. Quite some pressure can be applied, and it may even be a bit painful. However, the tissues should not be massaged or rubbed, as friction may delay wound healing or lead to dehiscence. Starting a fortnight after surgery, the patient should apply this pressure twice a day, in the morning and evening, for a period of about 4 weeks (Fig. 42).

The delicacy of the tissues requires the use of fine suture material. On the other hand, the considerable mechanical stress to which the area is subjected merely from walking or sitting, and normal everyday activities means that wound closure has to be as stable as possible. Delayed wound healing and wound dehiscence are the most common complications, especially with labial corrections. The patient must, of course, resume her normal activities as soon as she can, and this is usually possible within 2 or 3 days. The first 6 weeks represent a critical phase when any excessive strain should be avoided: no sexual intercourse, no jogging, horse riding, cycling, etc. during this time. If the patient really feels the need to exercise, after 2 weeks, she can use a cross trainer or stepper where there is a greater distance between the legs and no direct friction on the genital area.

Likewise, the use of tampons is not allowed for 6 weeks, especially after labia minora reduction, as the insertion of a tampon can tear the edges of the wound.

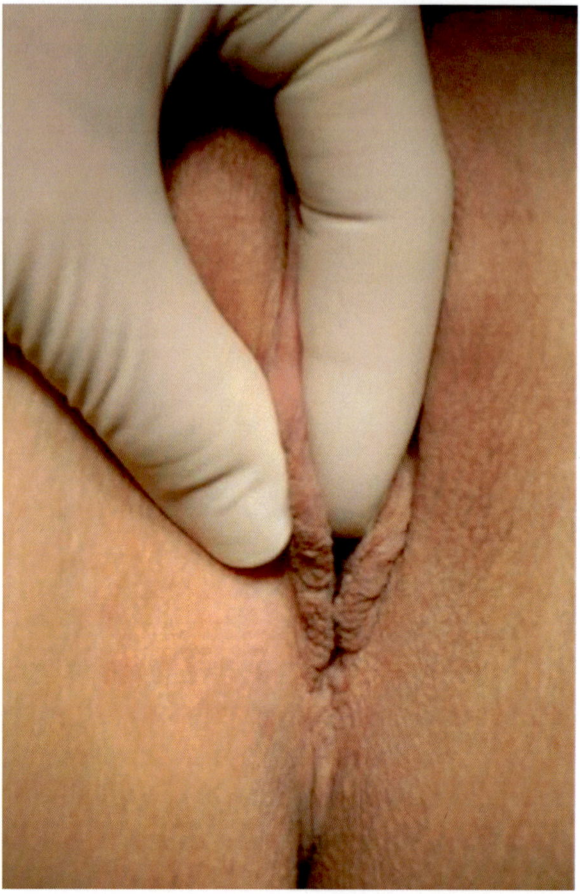

Fig. 42 Postoperative pressure with fingertips

Women should also not shave the genital area during this period, so as to avoid unnecessary manipulation.

Showers are allowed again after 2 days but without the use of soap or other cleansing agents for 1 week. It is not necessary to disinfect the area after the operation. Sitz baths soften the wound edges and are therefore not to be recommended.

As absorbable sutures have been used, there is no need to remove any stitches. Even so, as they are absorbed, the sutures may cause considerable itching. Should this happen, wound ointment, aloe vera gel, or even a cortisone cream can be applied. If they cause problems, the stitches can also be removed after about 10 days.

Pitfalls and Complications

Of the possible complications, delayed wound healing is statistically the most common. This is mainly because the genital region is under constant mechanical stress, even when sexual intercourse does not take place. Simply walking or sitting exerts forces on the edges of the wound and may prevent straightforward wound healing. Even so, the patient may carry out her normal everyday activities, always remembering to treat the area as gently as possible—no intense friction for 6 weeks after the operation, especially no sexual intercourse, cycling, jogging, etc.

The delicate tissues require the use of as fine a suture thread as possible, but the mechanical stresses on the area demand good stability. The best solution for wound closure is therefore to use 6–0 or 5–0 sutures placed at close intervals. A weak spot in the techniques described above is the point where the small lateral flap is inserted into the line of the labia minora. Wound dehiscence occasionally occurs here when the wound edges are not joined seamlessly, stably, and without tension (Fig. 43).

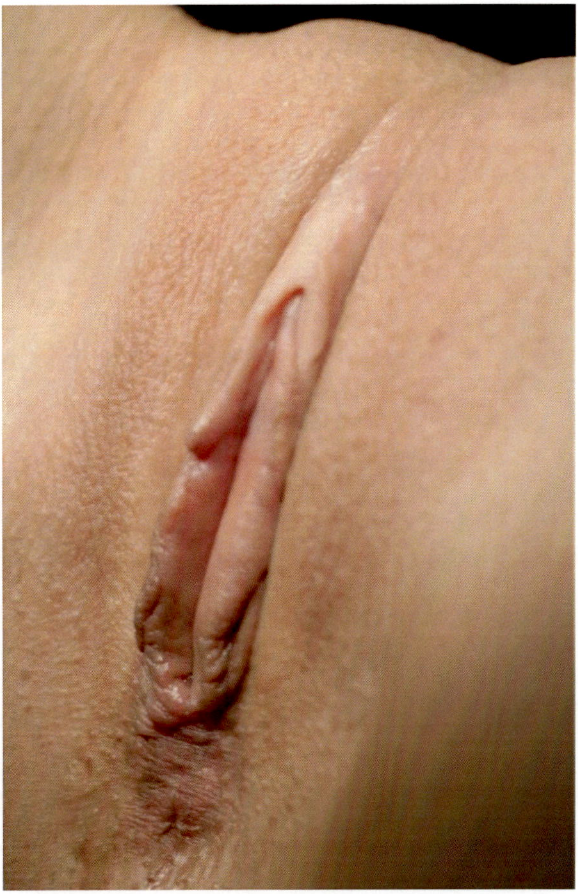

Fig. 43 Wound dehiscence with contour defect on the right labia minora

However, as the small flaps are under tension directed inferiorly in order to achieve effective downward tightening of the clitoral hood, these flaps should be anchored firmly and the skin largely relieved of tension.

Even when the resection lines are drawn identically on both sides and the surgeon achieves an optimal symmetry during the intervention, it is still possible for the two sides to heal differently in the postoperative period, leaving an asymmetry that can only be resolved with a corrective procedure. Possible reasons include unequal swelling, one side slipping beneath the other (which can be prevented by placing a gauze compress between the labia), unilateral postoperative bleeding, and different healing of the scars on the two sides.

Postoperative bleeding that requires revision surgery is very rare, but occurs particularly when the wound has been closed with a continuous subcutaneous suture. Small bleeds often occur after the patient has been to the toilet, but can be dealt with easily by applying direct pressure for few minutes.

Swelling always occurs, but to a variable extent. Up to 80% disappears within the first 6 weeks, the remainder resolves very slowly and can last for up to 6 months. Finger pressure applied as described above is the best method of preventing persistent swelling and ensuring optimal scar healing.

Sensory disturbances of the clitoris are usually irreversible and result in a diminished response to sexual stimulation and a reduced ability to orgasm. This needs to be prevented at all costs. Knowledge of the relevant anatomy and a gentle cautious approach, especially to the clitoral structures whenever it is necessary to touch them, are the key factors. Avoid excessive coagulation of any bleeding in the region of the clitoral shaft. Use only bipolar coagulation in this area.

It is possible that a sensitivity to touch develops along the line of the wound but this returns to normal with time. As a rule, however, the patient is unaware of this, as the genital area hurts and she will avoid touching it at first.

Alternative Techniques

For the sake of completeness, there are alternative labiaplasty techniques that have found their place in the literature for some time. The shared quality of all these methods is that they aim to reduce only the segment distal to the clitoris. These techniques do not include effective tightening or lifting of the clitoral hood, nor do they provide any correction of the prepuce or a protruding clitoris.

The only indication for these methods is isolated hypertrophy of the labia minora confined to the distal segment, and this finding is the exception rather than the rule.

The indication for these techniques is therefore limited, and, if they are used when there is hypertrophy of the entire labia, they not infrequently lead to an inharmonious appearance, resulting in a proximal segment that is too long and a distal segment that is often proportionately too short.

Technique According to G. Alter

Wedge resection is a relatively popular technique and is frequently used because it is not complicated to perform. A triangular section of the labium, with the apex pointing medially, is removed from below the clitoris. Closing the wound edges tightens and shortens the distal labial segment in a relatively short operating time. If too much tension is placed on the wound margins, however, there is often dehiscence and delayed wound healing (Fig. 44).

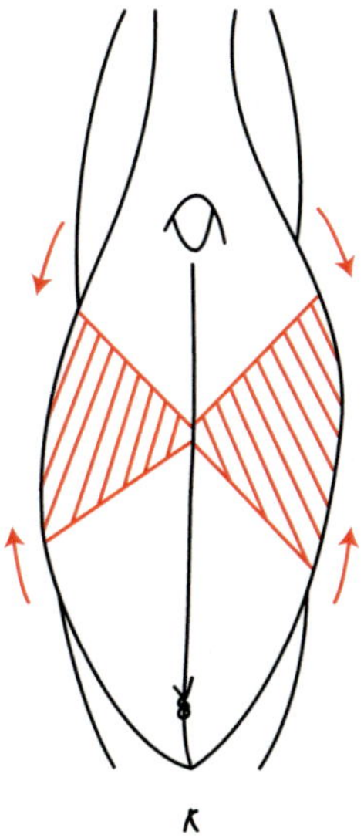

Fig. 44 Technique according to *G. Alter*

Technique According to C. Trichot

A wedge-shaped segment is resected at the lower labial pole, and the remaining part of the labia pulled downwards to tighten the tissues. When using this method, you have to be very careful that the vaginal introitus and the posterior commissure are reconstructed without tension and no scar or bridge of the skin develops, as this could be troublesome and painful during sexual intercourse (Fig. 45).

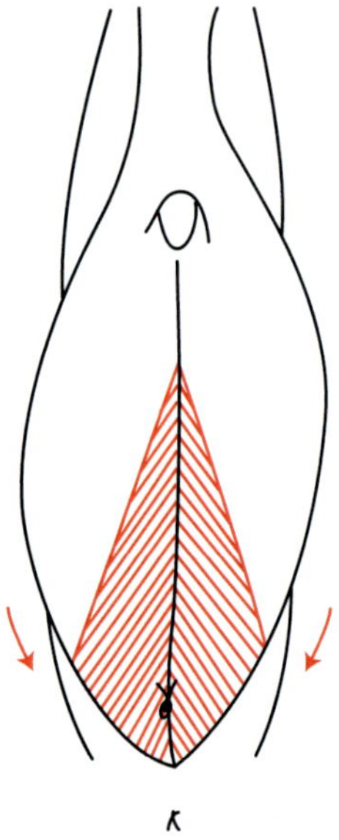

Fig. 45 Technique according to *C. Trichot*

Technique According to R. Rouzier

Here, a central segment is removed from the distal segment of the labia. The remainder is pulled inferiorly and fixed. Tightening of this part inferiorly, anchoring the labia in the region of the posterior commissure, may lead to distortion of the introitus if the tension on the distal labial segment is too great (Fig. 46).

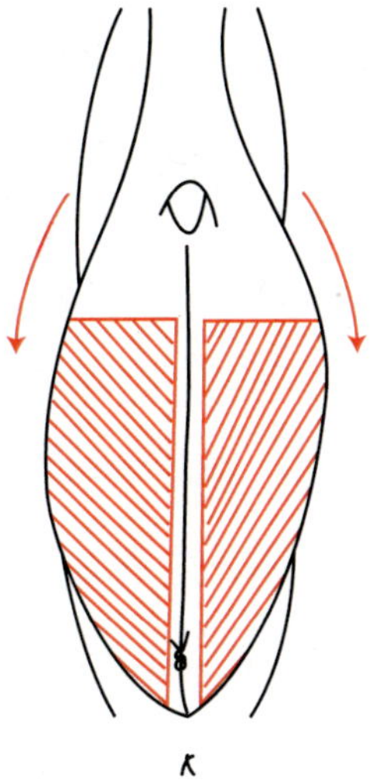

Fig. 46 Technique according to *R. Rouzier*

Technique According to H.Y. Choi

The removal of a central crescent-shaped segment allows moderate tightening in this labial segment (Fig. 47).

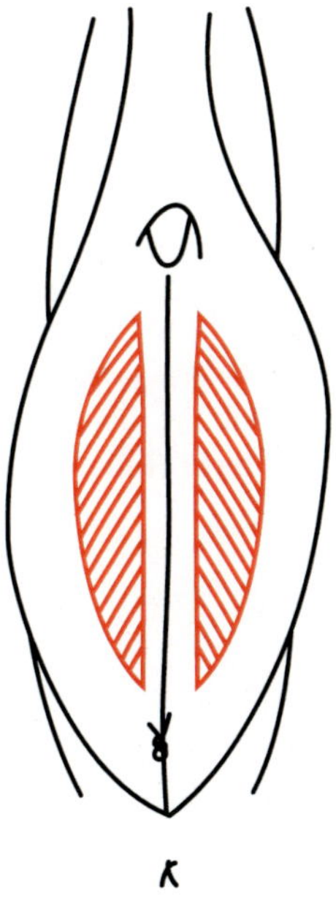

Fig. 47 Technique according to *H.Y. Choi*

Technique According to D. J. Hodgkinson

Reduction of this labial segment is achieved by resecting a strip of excess tissue along the free edge of the labium (Fig. 48).

Fig. 48 Technique according to *D.J. Hodgkinson*

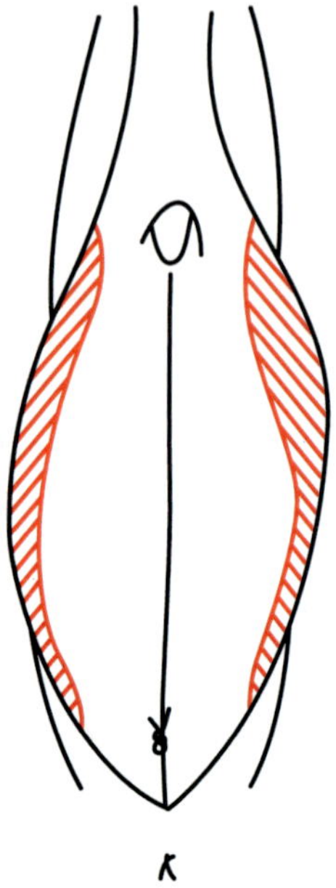

Technique According to S. M. Maas

Excess tissue is removed by a zig-zag excision along the free edge. The idea is to prevent the formation of a linear scar that would affect the stretch and elasticity of the labia. It is not necessary, however, since the labial skin is heavily folded, particularly in the distal segment, and is easily stretched despite any scar running along the free edge (Fig. 49).

Fig. 49 Technique according to *S.M. Maas*

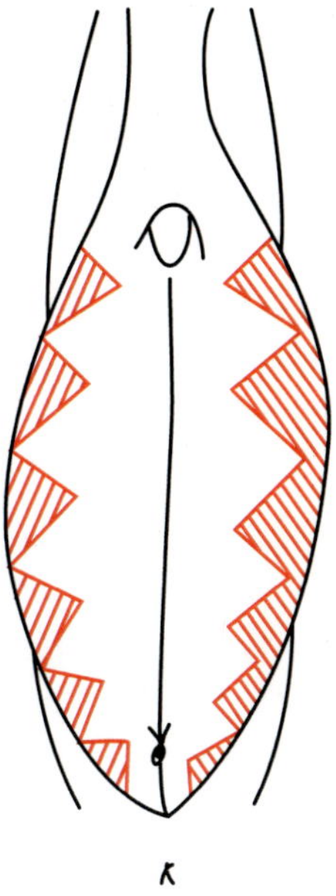

Technique According to F. Giraldo

A labial segment reminiscent of the shape of a church spire is removed somewhat below the clitoris (Fig. 50).

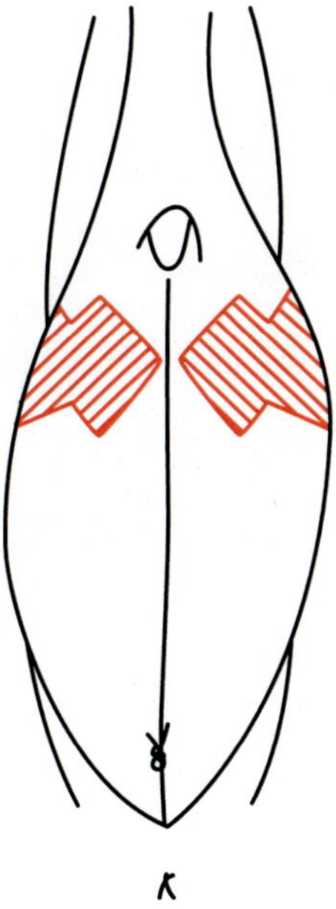

Fig. 50 Technique according to *F. Giraldo*

Labia Minora Reconstruction

Labial deformities are most often iatrogenic in nature. Fears of impairing the sensory innervation, mainly because of a lack of familiarity with the relevant anatomical detail, cause many surgeons to prefer labiaplasty in the segment of the labia minora below the clitoris. But as hypertrophy is usually also present in the clitoral hood and the prepuce, the result seems unbalanced when only the lower segment is corrected, giving the appearance of a microphallus that is even worse when there is clitoral protrusion. This is the most frequent deformity seen after labia minora reduction (Fig. 51a–d).

As most of the techniques reduce the labia minora only in the segment distal to the clitoris, this is also the area where most reconstructions are subsequently needed.

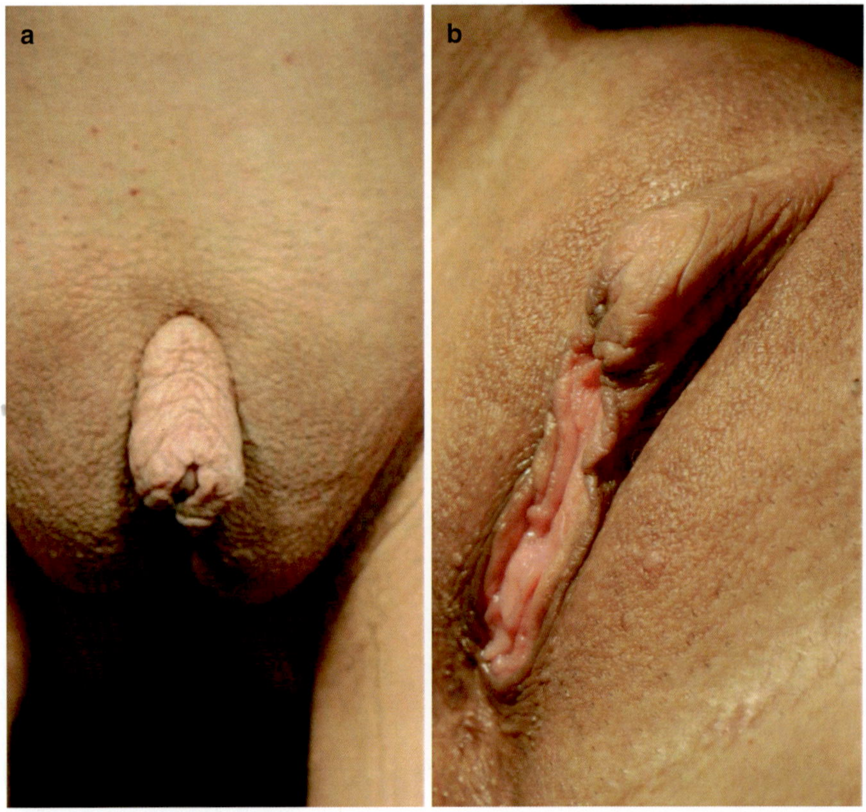

Fig. 51 (**a**) Unbalanced postoperative result after labia minora reduction only posterior to the clitoris leaving hypertrophy of the prepuce, the clitoral hood and the clitoral protrusion untreated. Frontal view, standing. (**b**) lithotomy position, oblique view. (**c**, **d**) another patient with the same deformity

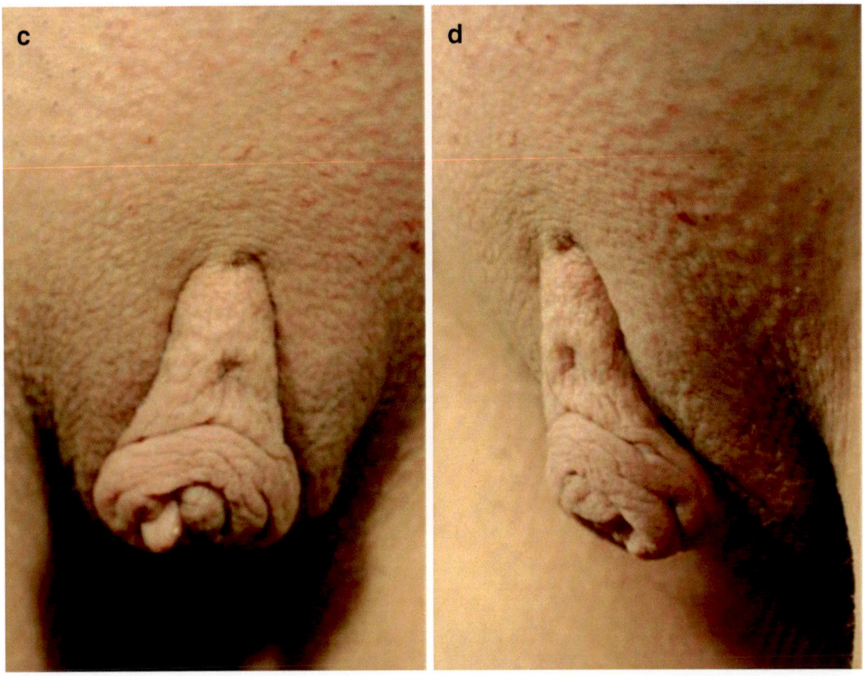

Fig. 51 (continued)

The problems include overresection with an almost complete lack of the labia minora, frayed edges, scarring, distortion, asymmetry, and considerable contour defects in this distal segment (Fig. 52a–g).

The excess tissue lying above can obviously be used to correct the distal segment. The operation, described by *G. Alter*, is the most appropriate for reconstructing overresection in the superior two-thirds of the distal labial segment. The surgical procedure is unfortunately at its limits for reconstruction of the inferior third of this segment, as the pedicle flap is often not long enough to reach the posterior commissure.

It is also possible to reconstruct the labial walls here using vaginal skin. But reconstructing the labia minora with vaginal skin should be viewed as a last resort in cases where there is no excess tissue in the proximal labial segment (prepuce). In addition, it is not possible to achieve any great labial height with this technique.

Skin grafts, of course, would be another option, but a skin graft is always aesthetically inferior to reconstruction with locoregional tissues. The colour and texture are not the same, nor is the graft sensitive, so I am not going to give any further details.

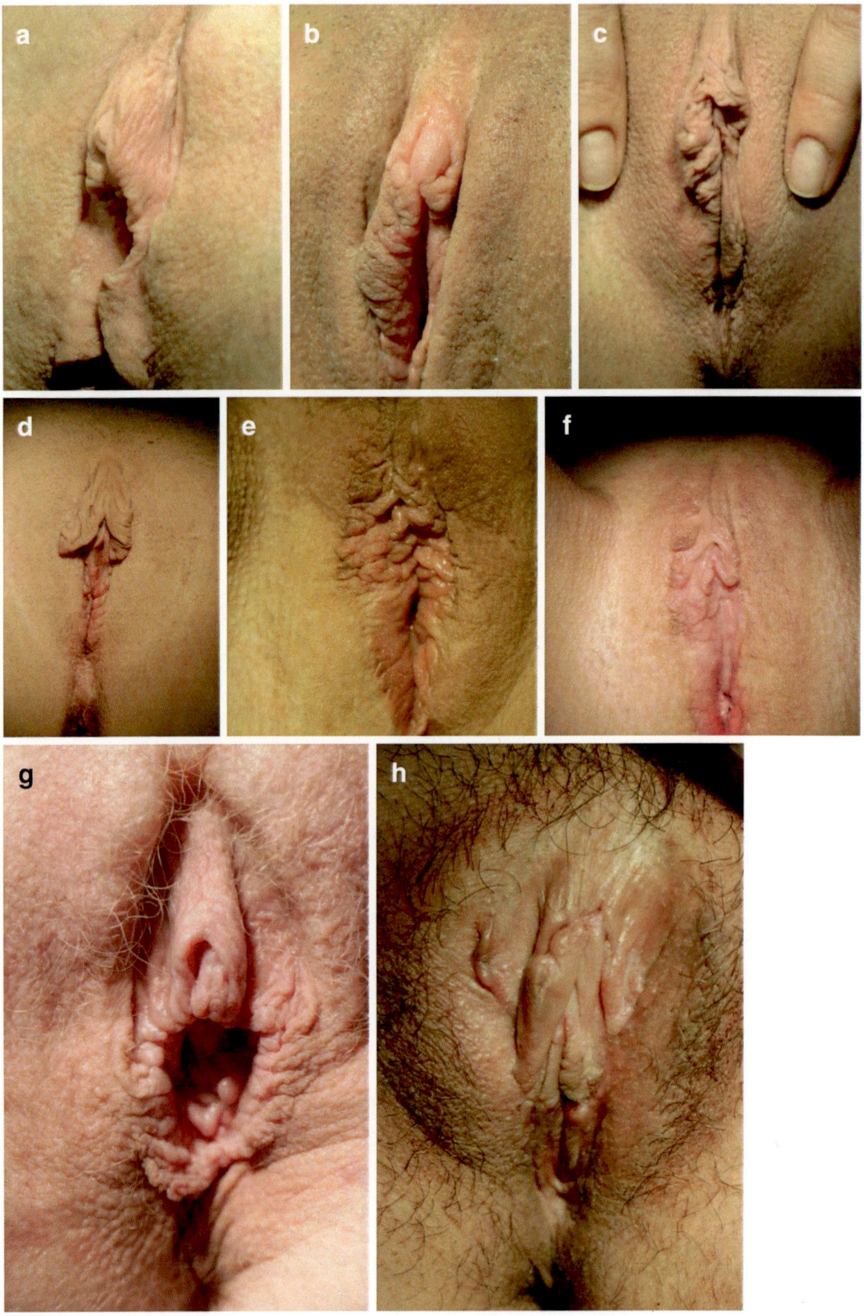

Fig. 52 Iatrogenic deformities following labiaplasty. (**a**) contour defect. (**b**) clitoral hood resection with total exposure of the glans. (**c**) asymmetry and partial over-resection. (**d**) undercorrection in the clitoral and preputial segment, inferior over-resection, frayed wound edges due to inappropriate skin closure. (**e-f**) amputation of the labia in the inferior segment, open introitus, frayed wound edges. (**g**) over-resection and asymmetry in the posterior segment, open vaginal entry. (**h**) complete distortion and partial labial amputation

Reconstruction with Lateral Prepuce Flaps

Indication

The labia minora is restored (Fig. 53a, b) in the segment below the clitoris by means of two distal pedicle flaps, consisting partly of the lateral prepuce and partly of the excess labial tissue above the clitoris. The vascular supply is ensured on the principle of a random pattern flap, since there is no defined axial vascular supply here. Even though the circulation in the genital region is very dense and allows a relatively narrow flap base, take care to create each flap to be as thick as possible, with the base as broad as possible, to prevent flap necrosis. This is all the more important, as the flap has to be rotated 180° downwards on its pedicle and sutured into place under slight tension.

Operation

Preparation corresponds to that for a *composite reduction labiaplasty*. In the distal segment, instead of drawing a resection level for the labial height, mark the line into which the flap will later be inserted. Residual labia to be used can be left and prepared; smooth out any frayed labial edges.

The areas of the skin marked on both sides of the middle of the shaft, whose tips extend into the origin of the interlabial folds, are not discarded as in a *CRL* but now form the flaps that will be used to replace the labia of the distal segment. Include a sufficiently thick subcutaneous layer in the dissection, directed as laterally as possible so as not to come too close to the branches of the dorsal nerve of the clitoris, which run towards the glans along the dorsum of the clitoral shaft at about 11 o'clock and 1 o'clock (Fig. 54).

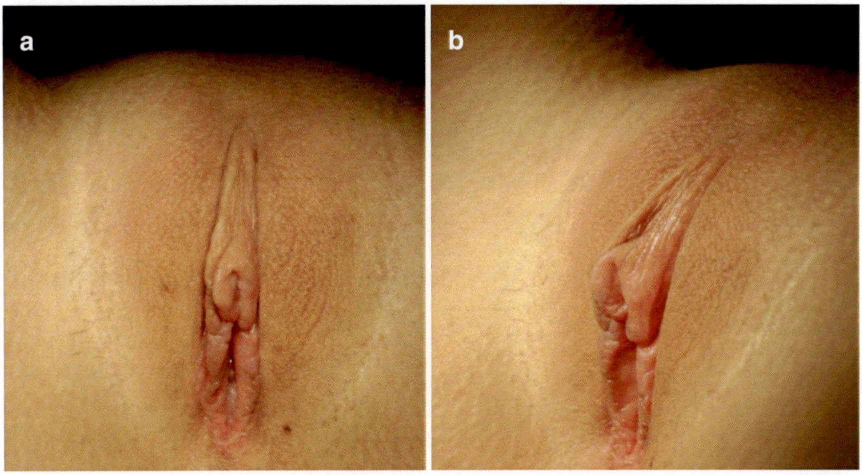

Fig. 53 (**a**) Iatrogenic deformation following labia redution plasty with overcorrection inferior to the clitoris and undercorrection above the clitoris. Reconstruction of the inferior part by lateral preputial flaps. Preoperative situation, frontal view, lithotomy position. (**b**) preoperative situation, oblique view, lithotomy position

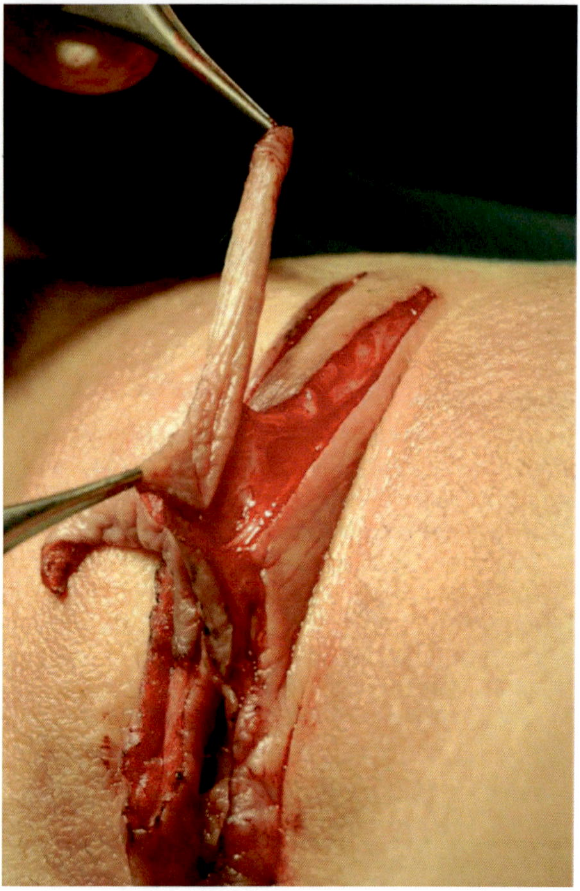

Fig. 54 raised lateral prepuce island—flap with inferior subcutaneous pedicle

Lateral flaps are also created along the distal clitoral hood as in a CRL. Pushing the clitoris distally, as when correcting clitoris protrusion, is also recommended in most cases, as the flap base will then reach further distally, making it easier to reconstruct the distal segment around the posterior commissure.

Once the flap has been lifted, it is rotated downwards (Fig. 55a–d) on its base and fixed subcutaneously with a 5–0 multifilament suture under slight tension to gain a longer reach. Close the wound with continuous 6–0 monofilament sutures along the inner and outer aspects of the labia (Fig. 56a–c).

Once the flap base has been turned, there may be an excess of the skin at the base of the flap. If it is necessary to remove part or all of this excess, do so as thinly as possible, so as not to reduce the width of the flap base.

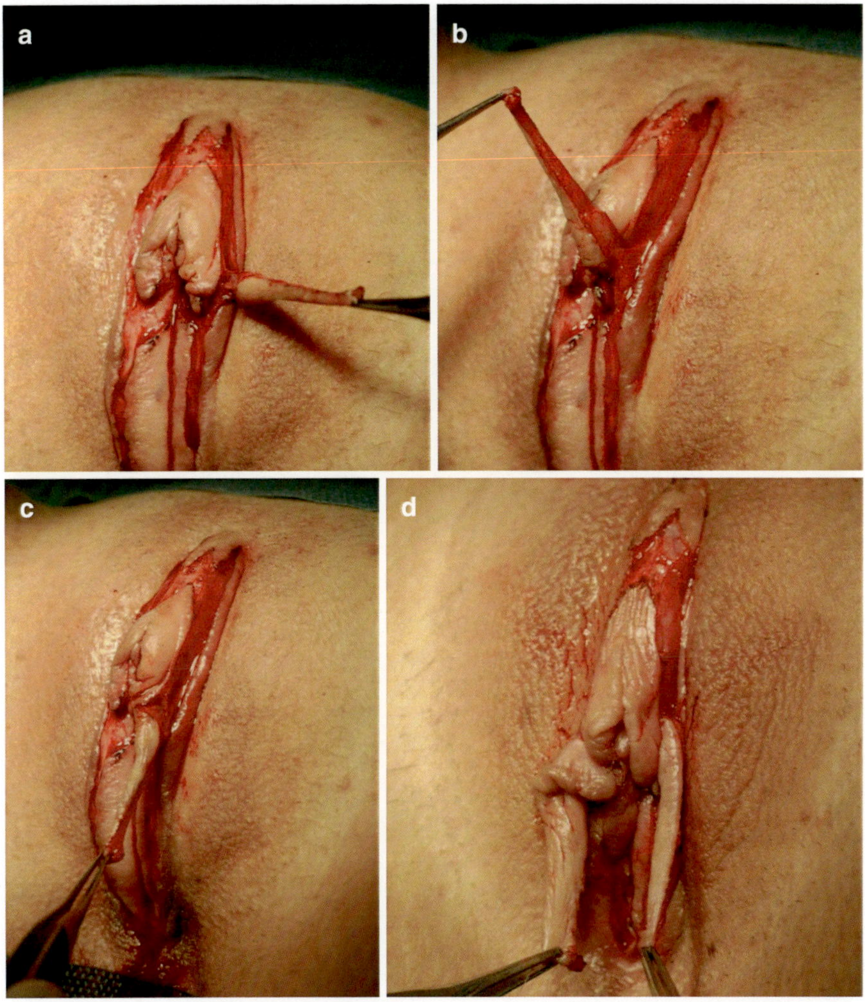

Fig. 55 (**a**) Rotating the flaps 180° (**a–d**)

Once the labia have been shaped and the wound closed, the reconstruction also requires through-and-through mattress sutures to be placed closely together through the labial walls to hold them erect. Do not place these sutures through the flap base or subcutaneous layer of the flap, so as not to compromise vascularisation.

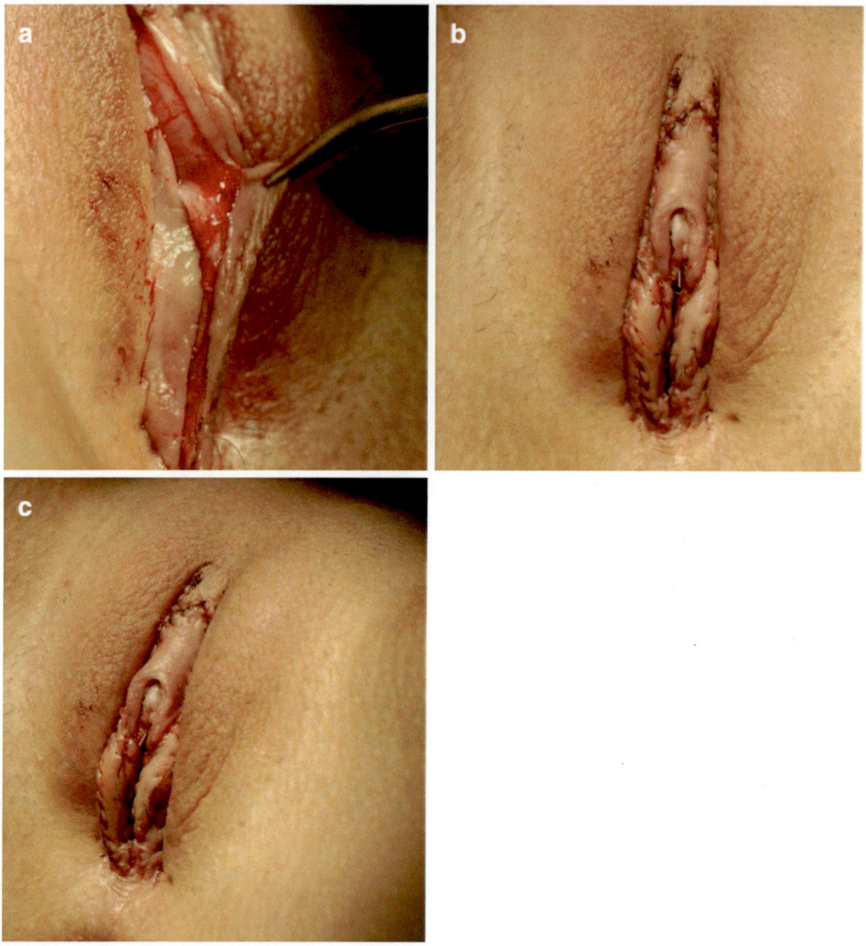

Fig. 56 (**a**) Inserting the flap under moderate tension, (**b**) Inserted flaps, frontal view, (**c**) inserted flaps, oblique view

Reconstruction with Vaginal Skin Advancement

Indication

Reconstruction of the labia with vaginal skin is the method of choice when there is no excess tissue above the clitoris, and a reconstruction according to *Alter* is no longer possible. This technique will not achieve any great labial height—some 5 to 7 mm at most (Fig. 57a, b).

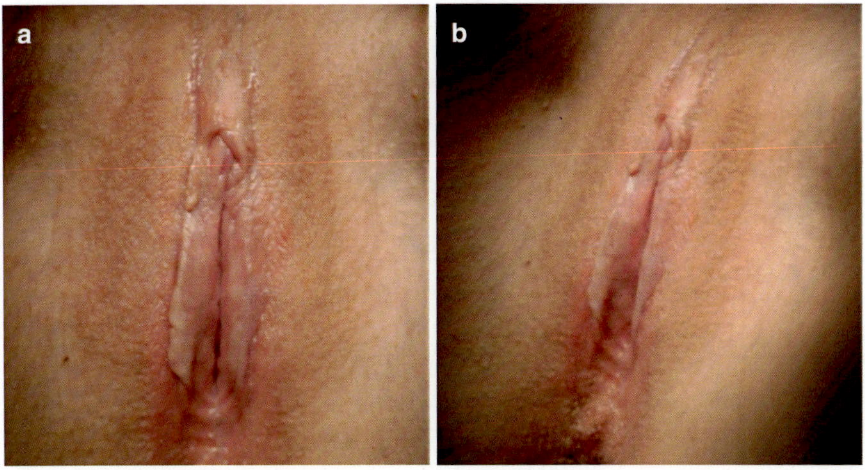

Fig. 57 (**a**) Iatrogenic deformation with labial over- resection superior and inferior to the clitoris frontal view, lithotomy position, (**b**) lateral view, lithotomy position

Fig. 58 Preoperative marking. *Dotted line* indicates the base of the labia at the interlabial fold

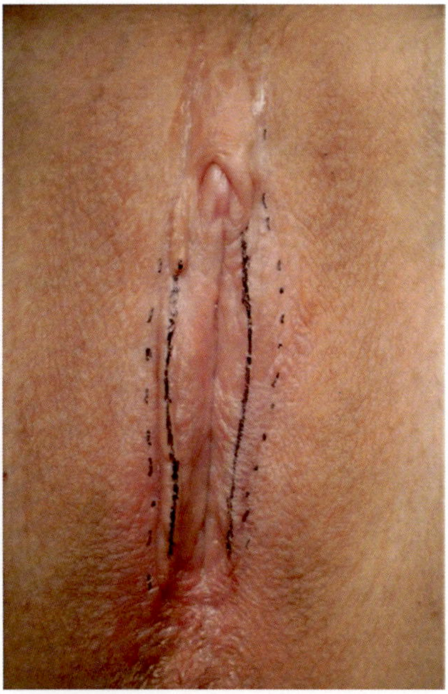

Operation

Draw in the incision lines for the planned operation (Fig. 58). In the region where the labia are to be reconstructed, the incision will follow the former line of the labial base, usually along the scar from the preceding labiaplasty. Using fine dissection scissors, detach the vaginal skin in the vestibule for about 2–3 cm. A radiosurgical device should not be used here, as there is a very high risk of perforating the vaginal skin by tangential dissection.

The skin is then detached lateral to the incision line as far as the interlabial fold, or even slightly further if necessary, and into the medial base of the outer labia. The width of this preparation is restricted by the start of the pubic hair, as otherwise the pubic hair would be shifted too far medially to the outer aspect of the labium minus (Fig. 59a–c).

Both the detached areas of the skin are then luxated upwards under tension, as bilateral advancement flaps, and fixed with a stronger 4–0 absorbable thread at the base of the flaps, using mattress sutures placed closely together (Fig. 60a–e). The two surfaces brought together in this way are then closed with a continuous mattress suture along the free edges using 6–0 multifilament thread.

To accentuate and strengthen the newly formed interlabial fold, the newly created labia are rotated laterally and fixed in this position on the inner aspects of the labia majora with percutaneous 6–0 absorbable sutures (Fig. 61a, b).

During postoperative healing, the labia have the tendency to flatten and sometimes spread out entirely. Together with the limited labial height, this is one of the weaknesses of the method. To prevent this from happening, it is absolutely necessary for the patient to squeeze the labia as described previously, starting after about 2 weeks, in order to maintain the height of the labia (Fig. 62a, b).

It is, of course, also possible to combine the two procedures. If a vaginal skin reconstruction is performed together with the lateral prepuce flaps, a greater labial height will be achieved, as the results of the two procedures are additive.

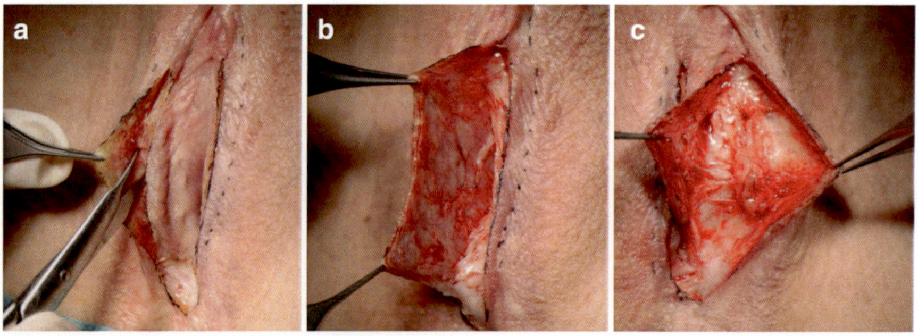

Fig. 59 (**a**) Lateral undermining including skin of the labia majora, right side, (**b**) Medial undermining including vaginal skin, left side, (**c**) Medial and lateral skin advancement, left side

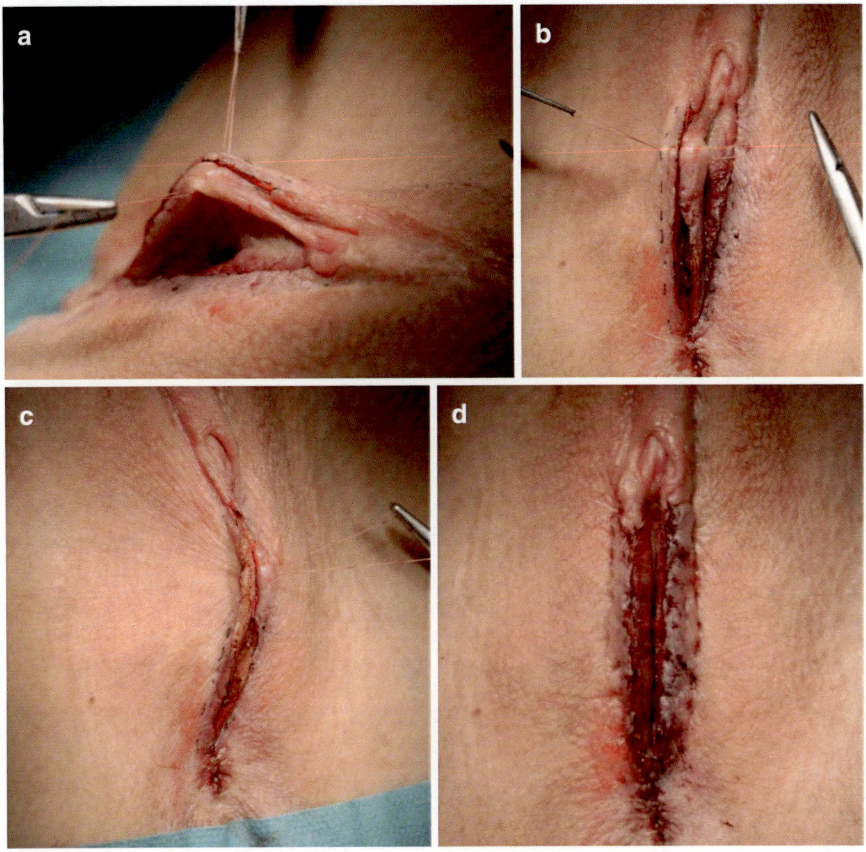

Fig. 60 (**a**) Mattress sutures forming the labia minora, medial view, (**b**) mattress sutures erecting the labia minora, frontal view, (**c**) the position of the mattress sutures determines the new interlabial fold, lateral view, (**d**) mattress sutures along the entire labial length, (**e**) newly formed labia minora

Fig. 60 (continued)

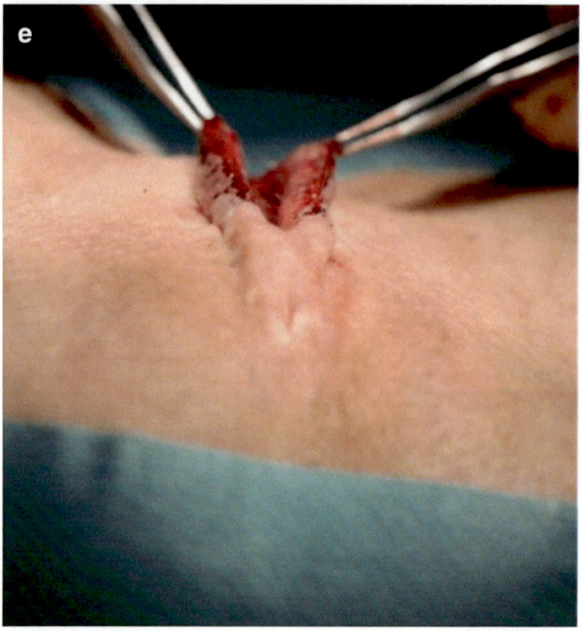

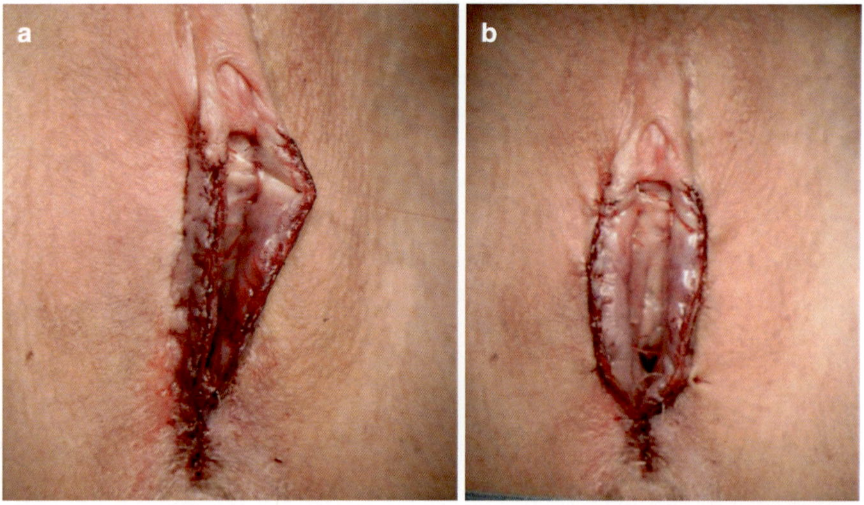

Fig. 61 (**a**, **b**) Attaching the labia minora to the labia majora to countour the new interlabial fold

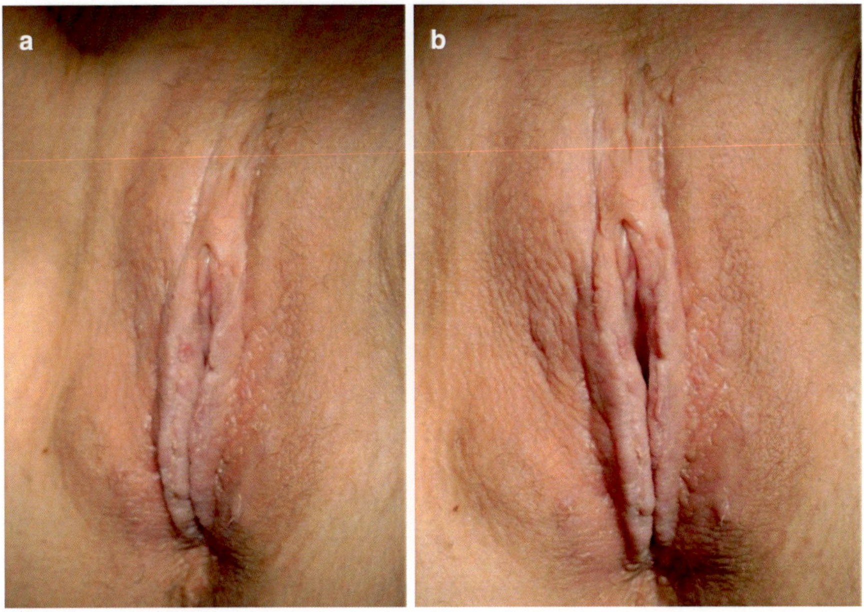

Fig. 62 (**a**) Situation 4 weeks after surgery, lateral view, lithotomy position. (**b**) Frontal view, lithotomy position

Examples
Patient 1
Labia reconstruction with lateral perpuce-flaps

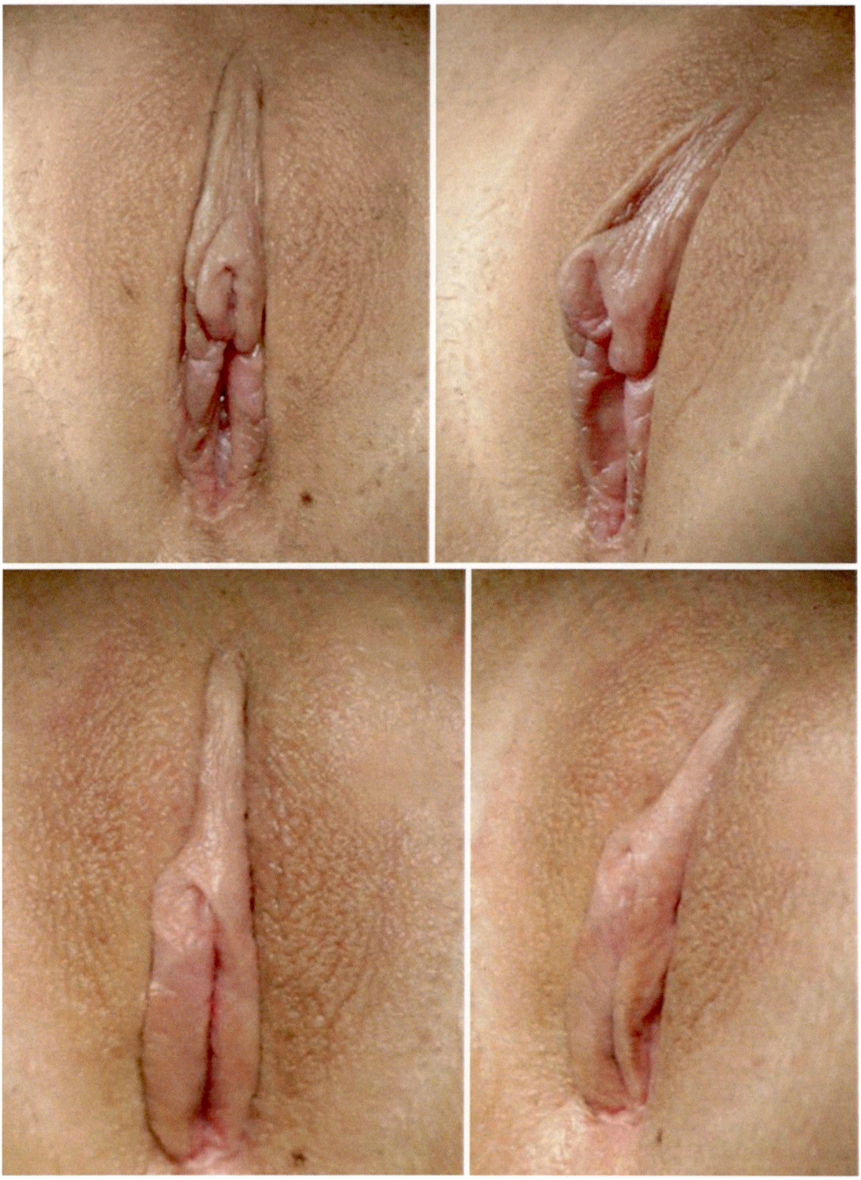

Patient 2
Labia reconstruction with lateral prepuce-flaps
Pre-, intra-, immediate post-OP and long term post-OP

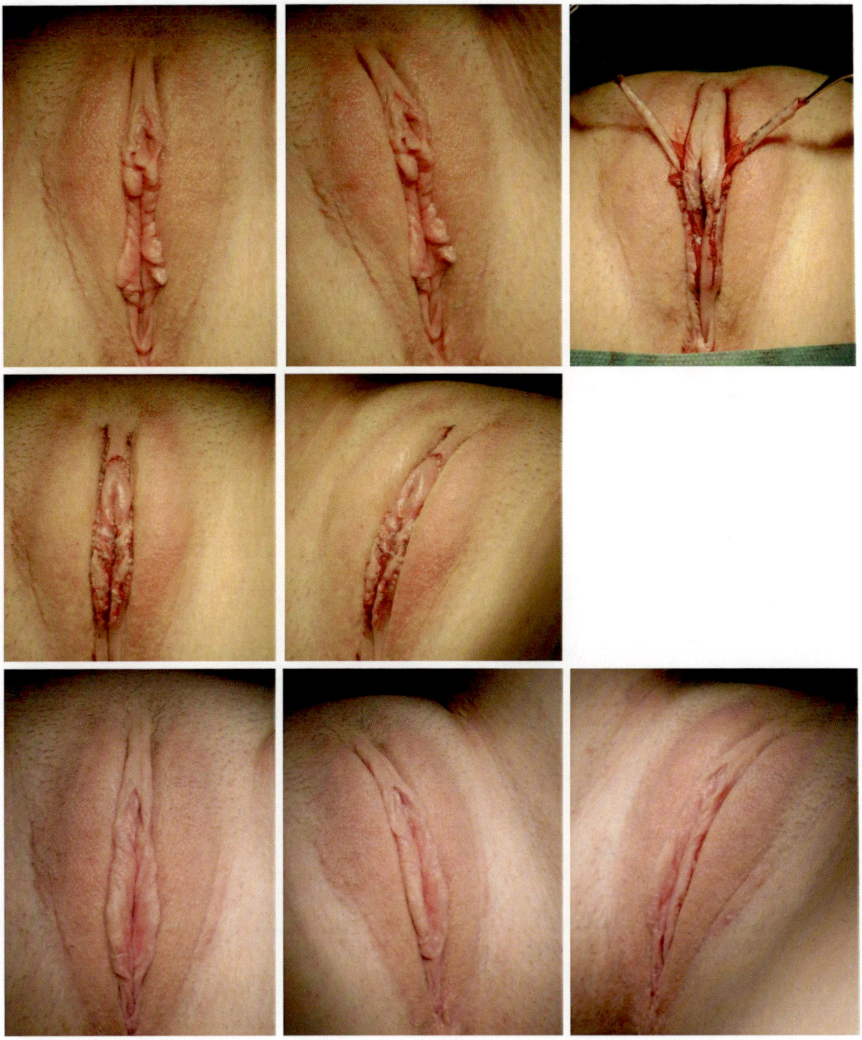

Patient 3
Labia reconstruction with vaginal skin advancement

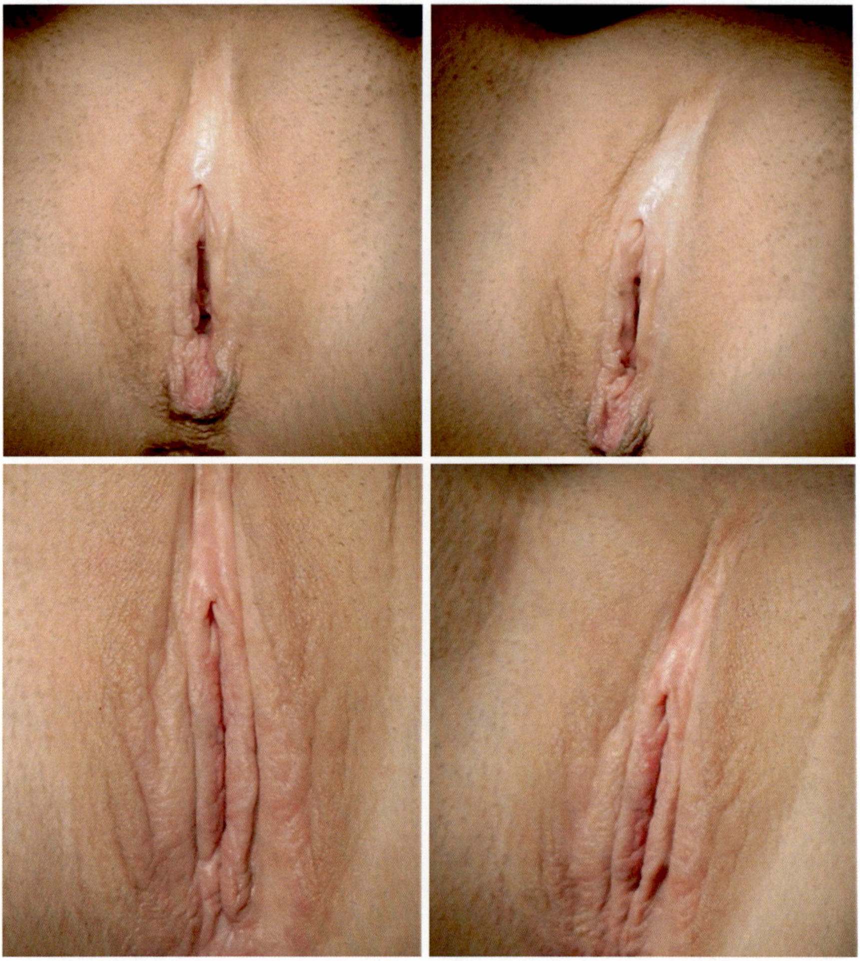

Patient 4
Labia reconstruction with lateral perpuce-flaps

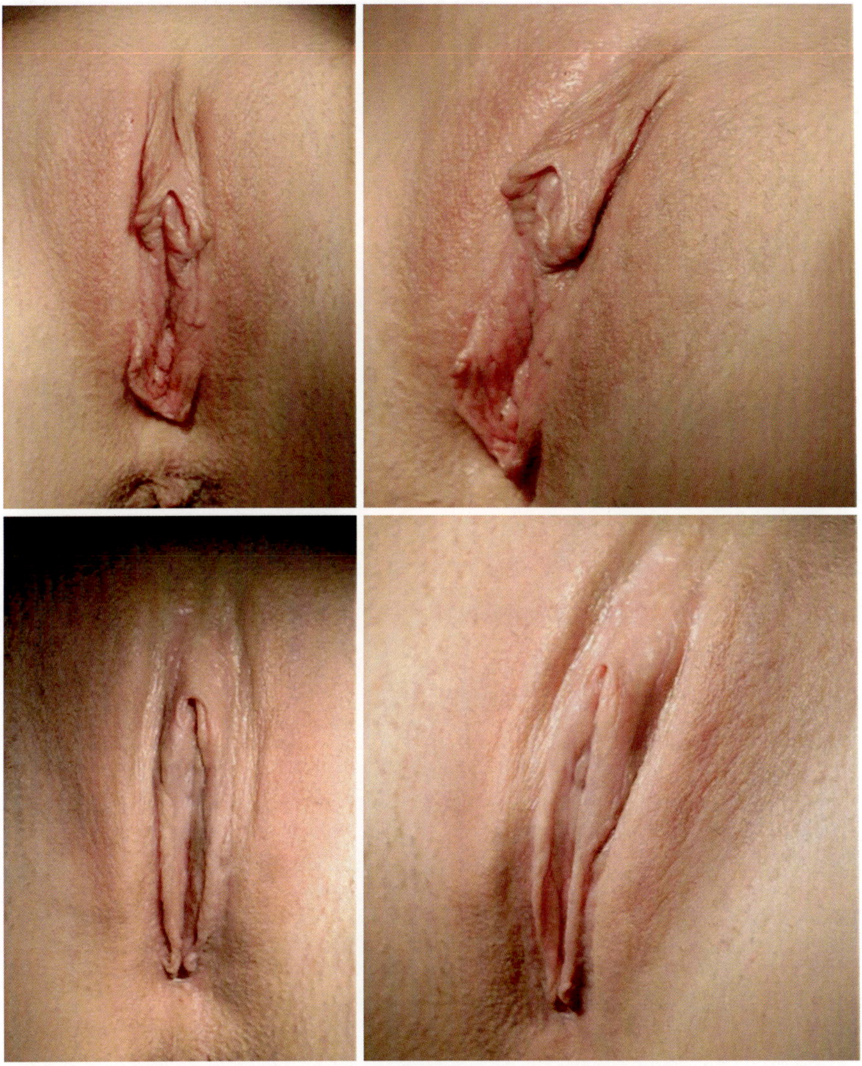

Patient 5
Labia reconstruction with lateral prepuce-flaps and vaginal skin advancement

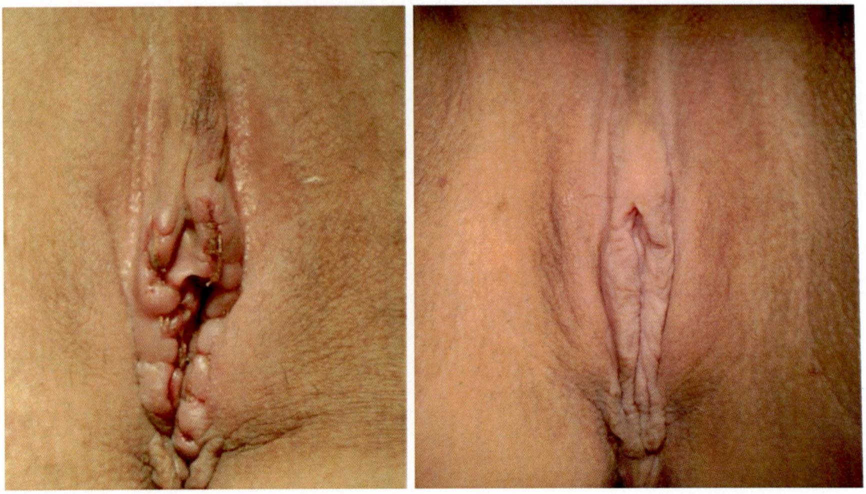

Patient 6
Labia reconstruction with lateral prepuce-flaps and vaginal skin advancement

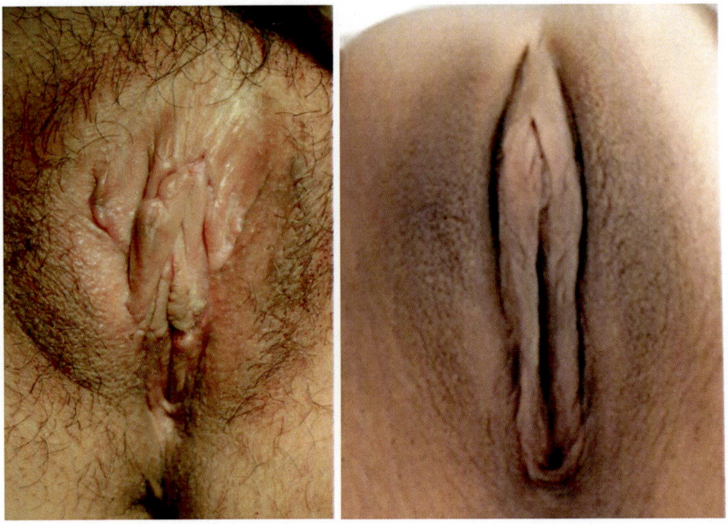

Labia Majora

The shape and consistency of the labia majora change considerably with age. In childhood and adolescence, the labia are rather firm thanks to the abundant fatty tissue over which the skin is firmly stretched (Fig. 1).

Young women do not show a great variation in the shape of the labia majora, certainly not to the extent of the variation found with the inner labia. But as women age, their individual differences become visibly more pronounced. The fat atrophy in various regions of the body that invariably comes with age may be particularly noticeable in the labia majora, and when there is also sagging and excess labial skin (analogous to the hypertrophy and sagging of the scrotal skin in men), the labia majora hang down as empty skinfolds. Not only is this aesthetically unattractive but it may also cause functional problems: mechanical protection and vaginal closure

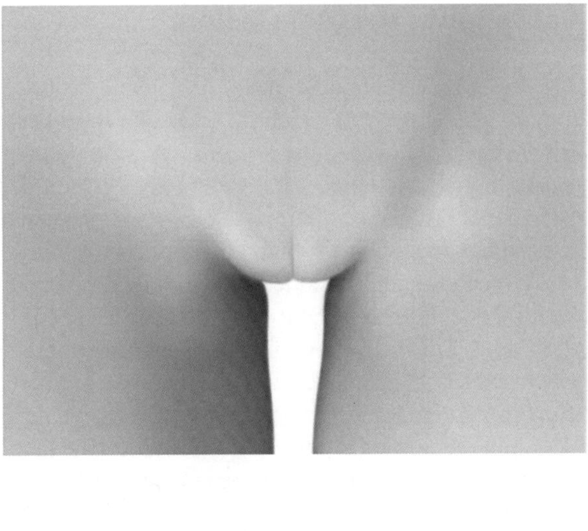

Fig. 1 "Ideal appearance" of the labia majora

S. Gress, *Aesthetic and Functional Labiaplasty*,
DOI 10.1007/978-3-319-60222-6_4

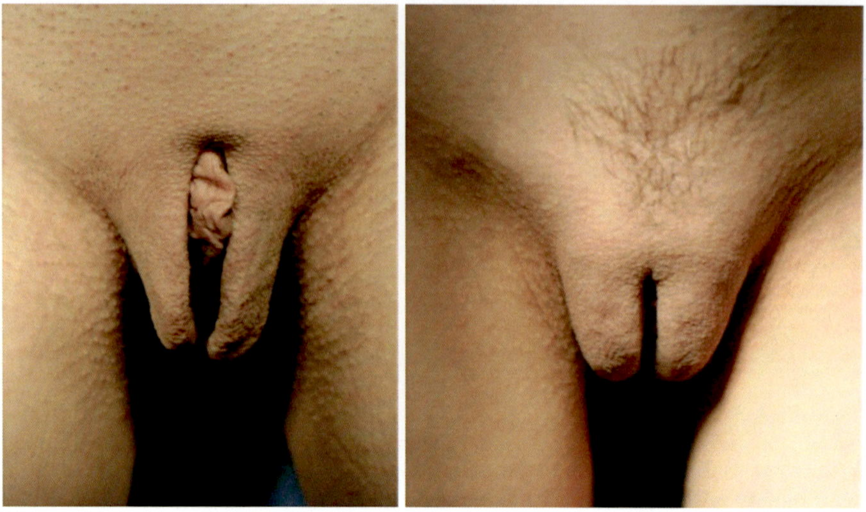

Fig. 2 Ageing labia majora with skin excess and loss of volume due to fat atrophy

functions are lost, so that dryness, inflammation, and candida infections are encountered more frequently (Fig. 2).

Treatment is derived from the following observations:

If there is fat atrophy, volume replacement with autologous fat is indicated. If there is excess labial skin, the labia majora require tightening. Since the two conditions generally coexist, the best solution is to combine both therapeutic options.

Reduction of the Labia Majora

The difficulty in reducing/tightening the labia majora is that there is no defined anatomical anchor point to which skin tension can be fixed and maintained. If too much labial skin is removed, there is distortion and/or gaping of the vaginal introitus. This must definitely be avoided. It is better to err on the side of caution and ensure that the wound margins can be approximated without tension once the excess skin has been removed. Although this sounds easy in theory, it is not so easy in practice.

The scars should be hidden and be as inconspicuous as possible, and the tightening of the labial skin should be as efficient as possible. The anatomy of the region does not leave many possibilities open, however, since the scars cannot lie anywhere except in the interlabial fold. Scars running directly on the backs of the labia, even in zigzags, are obsolete, as these scars would always be visible. One other possibility would be to make the incision on the lateral origin of the labia majora, close to the genitofemoral sulcus, but here, too, the scar would be very noticeable, similar to an inner thigh lift. The only remaining option is an incision in the interlabial fold, resecting excess skin from there and, in principle, tightening the structures in an inferomedial direction.

Another point to consider in the preoperative planning is the height of the inner labia. A reduction in the labia majora may cause the labia minora to protrude beyond their cover and become more visible than before the operation. Warn the patient in advance if this is to be expected.

Operation

Take measurements of the excess tissue with the patient standing but mark the incision lines with the patient in the lithotomy position. The spindle-shaped resection figure lies with one side along the interlabial fold except for the superior segment: at this point, i.e. along the clitoral shaft, the incision should run somewhat lateral to the interlabial fold, at a distance of about 2–3 mm, in order to maintain the curve of the medial origin of the labia majora.

The width of the spindle corresponds to the element of tightening: depending on the extent of the hyperplasia, it is between 1 and 2 cm, sometimes even more. The maximum width of the spindle is sited in the longitudinal middle of the outer labia, a little below the glans clitoris. The excess tissue is best excised with the high frequency unit (Fig. 3a, b).

Afterwards, the wound margins should largely lie together or deviate from each other only slightly (Fig. 4). This is most important for tension-free wound closure. To allow a relaxed skin closure, subcutaneously mobilise the labial skin about 1 cm laterally. Use 4-0 absorbable sutures with an over-and-over technique for the subcutaneous wound closure. This reduces the risk of postoperative bleeding and increases the consistency of the labia by gathering the subcutaneous tissues.

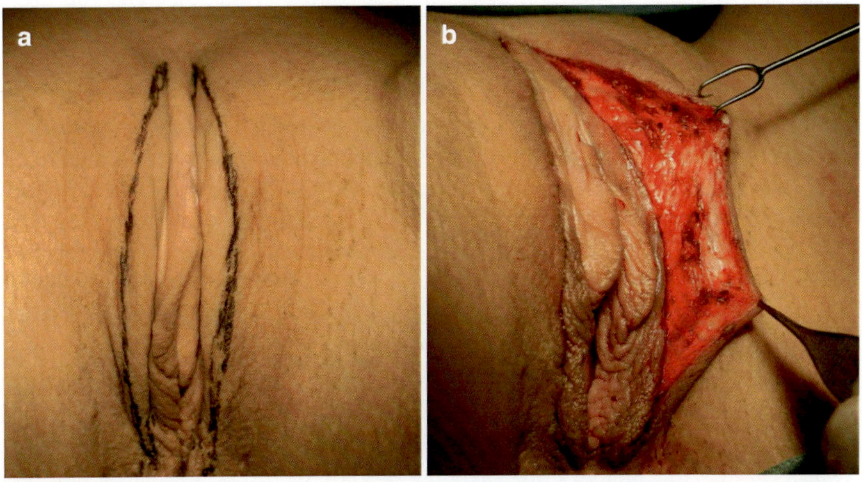

Fig. 3 (**a**) Marked spindle of labia majora skin to be removed, lithotomy position, frontal view. (**b**) Situation after skin excision, lithotomy position, oblique view

Fig. 4 No significant deviation of wound edges after skin removal

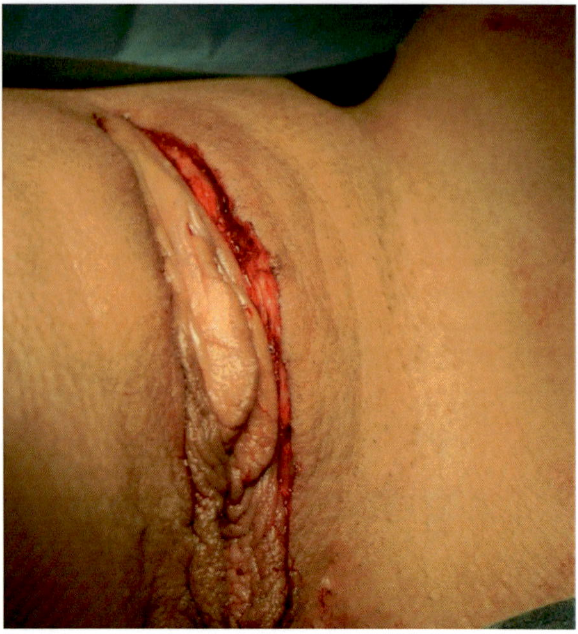

The skin is tightened obliquely downwards, in a slightly inferomedial direction towards the perineum, to direct the pull-away from the vaginal vestibule and the vaginal introitus.

When the findings show extensive changes, a back cut can be made at the origin of the labia majora, directed laterally from the posterior commissure, and after excising a triangle of the inferior labial skin (*Burow triangle*), tightening in an almost vertical direction will achieve an increased effect (Fig. 5a–d).

Use a running suture with a 5-0 absorbable monofilament thread for skin closure. As a rule, intradermal suturing techniques are not advisable in labial surgery, as they withstand mechanical stresses less well than over-and-over continuous skin sutures. An exception should be made, however, in the superior part of a labia majora reduction, i.e. parallel to the clitoral shaft, and an intradermal suture used to close the skin in this segment. This will prevent needle entry and exit sites being visible later on.

Tightening of the labia majora causes tension on the inner labia. If the labia minora have little height, they may become too flat. This does not change after the swelling has gone down and the wound has healed, that is to say, the original height of the labia minora is not spontaneously restored but remains what it has become.

In order to guard against or prevent this, maintain the height of the inner labia by taking the bites of the continuous skin suture through the base of the labia minora at regular intervals in the area distal to the clitoris; this will prevent the inner and outer aspects of the labia minora from spreading (Fig. 6).

The patient should place gauze compresses between the labia minora for 2 weeks after surgery, in order to maintain the position and height of the labia minora.

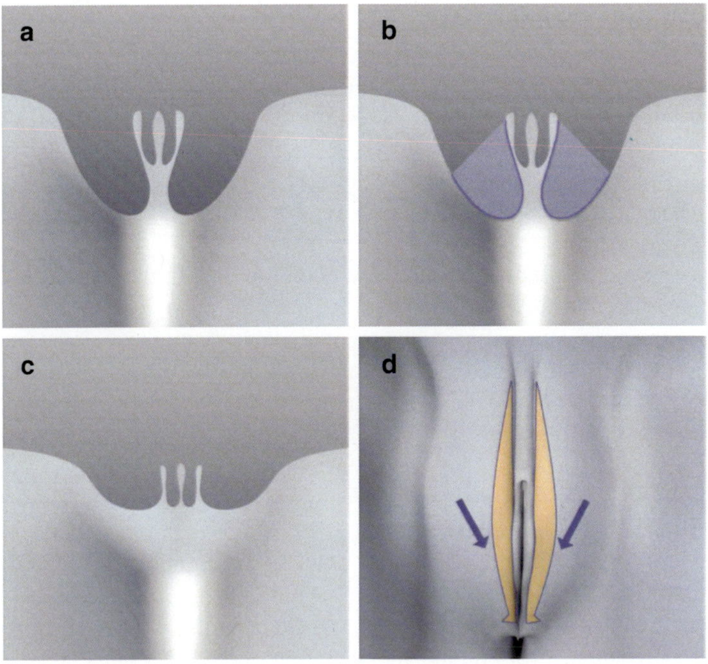

Fig. 5 (**a**) Hypertrophy of the labia majora, frontal view standing. (**b**) Marking of tissue to be removed, frontal view standing. (**c**) Situation after resection of tissue excess, frontal view standing. (**d**) Labia excess is removed (*yellow area*) and wound closure is performed under inferior oblique tension. Optionally *Burow's triangles* can be excised at the posterior commissure, frontal view, lithotomy position

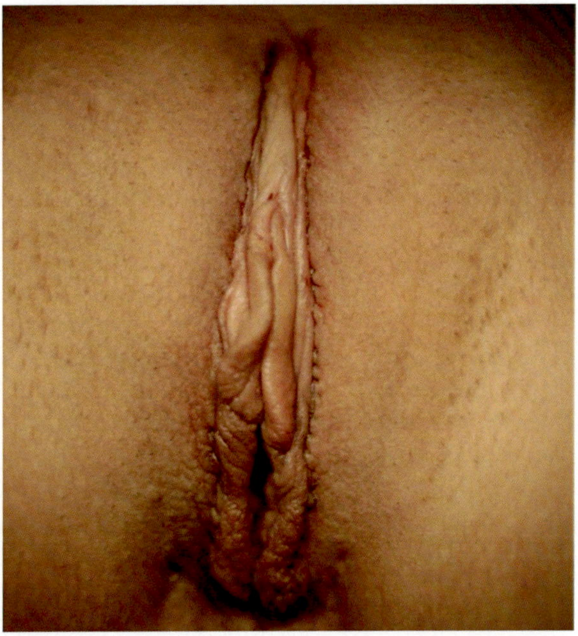

Fig. 6 Situation after wound closure, lithotomy position, frontal view

Postoperative Management

Postoperative care of a reduction labiaplasty of the labia majora is somewhat less complicated than after labia minora reduction. After a period of 2 weeks, the patient can also apply fingertip pressure along the line of the scar to promote healing and obtain an optimal scar. Special scar creams can also be used.

Sexual intercourse is allowed again after 4 weeks, as is jogging, cycling, horse riding, etc.

Tampons can be used at any time. To avoid pulling on the scar, it is, however, advisable to treat the area gently and not to shave the pubic hair.

Postoperative swelling after reduction of the labia majora goes down very slowly and may take up to 1 year. It is important to inform the patient about this before surgery, as swelling of the outer labia is more pronounced than swelling of the inner labia and questions often arise.

Volume Filling (Lipostructure)

As the fatty tissue in the labia majora diminishes with age, it makes sense to fill the void with autologous fat. Absorbable alloplastic materials, such as hyaluronic acid, are not really suitable for volume augmentation of the outer labia, as they usually become encapsulated and indurated. In addition, a large volume is required, which becomes expensive. The use of non-absorbable alloplastic materials is obsolete, as these materials may cause unpredictable late complications, e.g. chronic inflammatory reactions, induration, etc., which can only be treated by surgical intervention.

The method of choice is volume augmentation by autologous fat transfer, also called fatgrafting or lipostructure. This method, popularised by *S. Coleman*, has been well established for many years, and fat grafting is now used for volume augmentation in all areas of the body. The fat cells transferred survive long term whenever they connect with blood vessels that supply oxygen and nutrients. The cells obtain their nutrition by diffusion for the first few days, but then capillaries should develop. If no blood supply is established, the fat cells die and are resorbed into the body.

The survival rate of the fatty tissue depends on multiple factors. The key issues are the blood supply of the graft site, the donor site, the way in which the fat cells are prepared, the way in which the fat transfer is performed, the quantity of fatty tissue per volume unit of the graft site, patient care after the procedure, etc.

It is not expected that a high percentage of the fat transferred will survive in the labia majora. To date, there are no quantitative studies, but estimates based on clinical observation reckon that the survival rate is only about 30–40%. This fact should certainly be taken into consideration when planning the operation. The most common complication of fat grafting is undercorrection—overcorrection is not very likely.

Operation

The inner aspect of the knee and the outer aspect of the thigh are both suitable donor sites (Fig. 7). First of all, the donor and graft sites are marked and injected with local

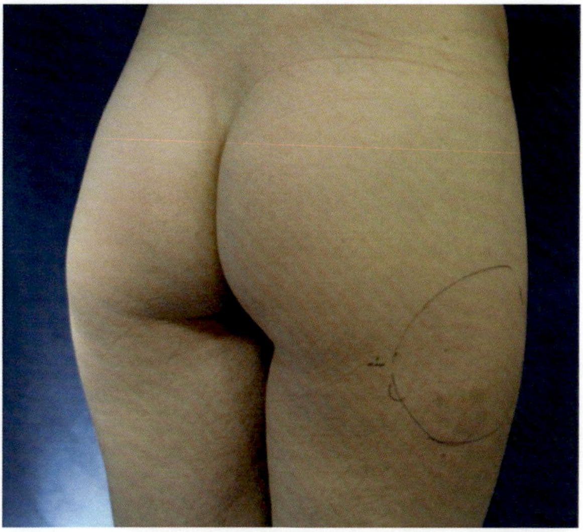

Fig. 7 Suitable donor site: the lateral thighs

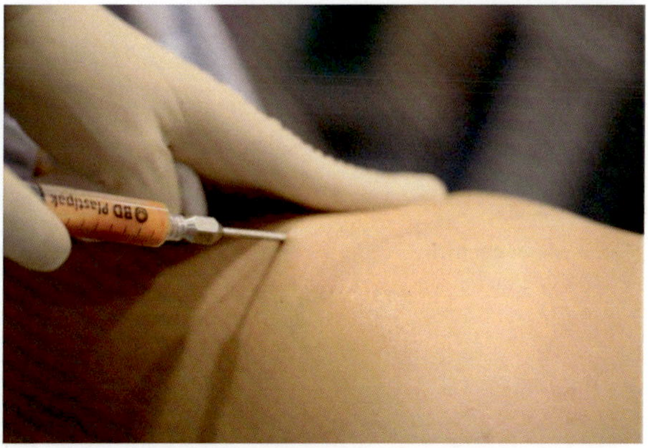

Fig. 8 Harvesting autologous fat

anaesthetic and Suprarenin [adrenaline]. After waiting a few minutes for the anaesthetic to take effect, remove fatty tissue through a stab incision with a special cannula. Attach the cannula to the Luer lock fitting of a 10 mL syringe, withdraw the plunger until resistance is felt, and then advance the cannula into the donor site. Remove the fat with fan-like movements, but avoid working too superficially; otherwise dimples may form (Fig. 8).

Centrifuge the harvested fat at about 3000 rpm for approximately a minute. When the syringe is removed from the centrifuge, three phases can be distinguished: the lowest phase is red and consists of blood and the injected solution. The middle phase is white/yellow and consists of the fatty tissue that will be used for the graft. The uppermost phase is oily and contains disrupted fat cells (Fig. 9).

Discard the lowest and uppermost phases and fill the middle phase into a 1 mL Luer lock syringe.

The fatty tissue is then ready for transfer. It can be injected into the labia majora using either a blunt cannula or one with a sharp tip (Fig. 10a, b). In doing so, it is

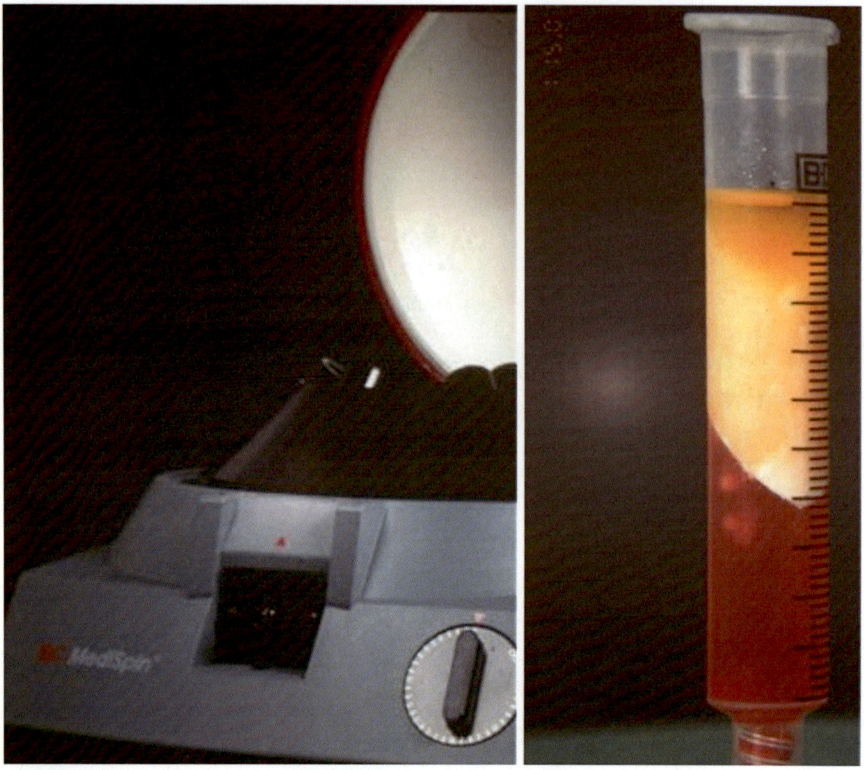

Fig. 9 After centrifuging, the harvested fat seen in the middle phase contains the fat cells suitable for transplantation

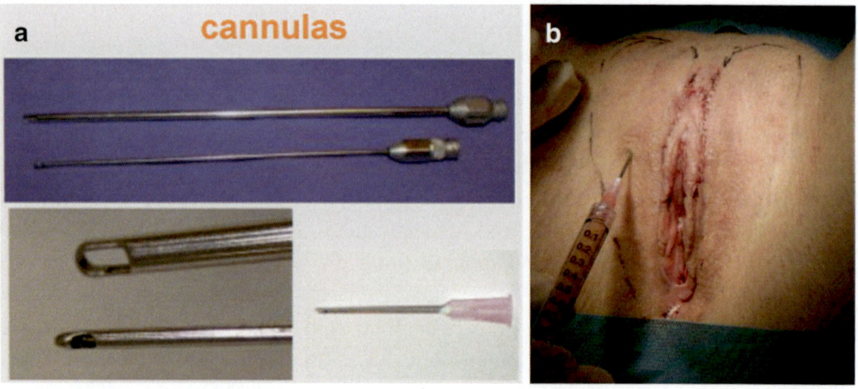

Fig. 10 (**a**) Cannulas for harvesting and injecting fat. (**b**) Fat injection with a sharp needle

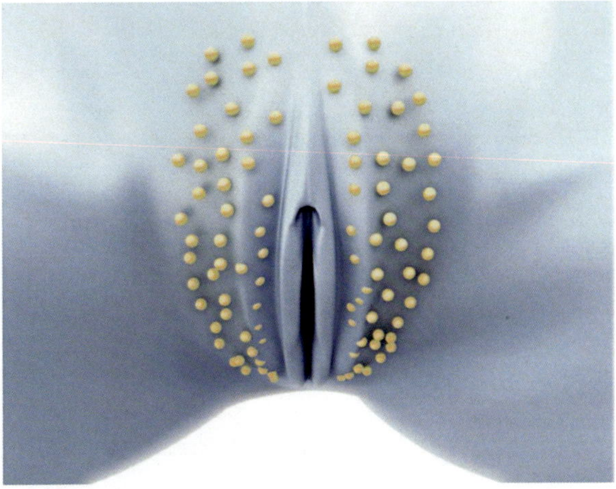

Fig. 11 Three-dimensional distribution of the transplanted fat parcels

important that the fat comes to lie in the recipient site as thin ribbons or isolated punctate grafts in different levels, also superficially. Capillaries forming the vascular supply can extend over a maximum distance of 3 mm. If a large clump of fatty tissue is injected, the capillaries have no chance of reaching the inside of the graft: the fat cells there will die and be resorbed. Oil cysts can also develop. It is therefore important to distribute the fat cells diffusely over a three-dimensional space at the graft site to give them the best chance of establishing a blood supply and survival (Fig. 11).

As mentioned previously, the main problem is that the survival rate of the transferred fat is not very high, being only about 30% in the labia majora. Considerable overcorrection is therefore always recommended. Depending on requirements, some 20–40 mL, or even more, can be injected into each outer labium (Fig. 12a–e).

Postoperative Management

After autologous fat transfer, the patient should largely avoid pressure on the labial area. If at all possible, she should not sit on it during the 14 days immediately following the procedure. Antibiotic cover is advisable. The injected fatty tissue may become encapsulated and can be felt as small indurated areas. They are, however, usually only temporary and can be resolved with gentle pressure or massage.

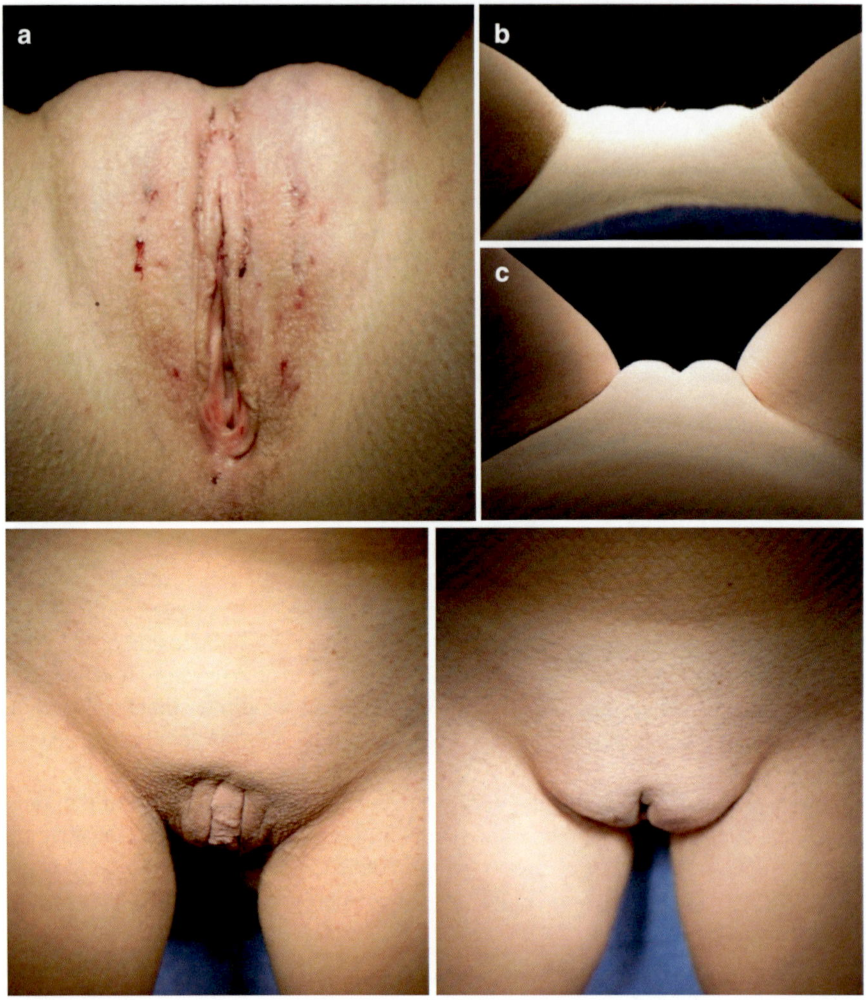

Fig. 12 (**a**) Labia majora augmentation with fat injection, lithotomy position, frontal view. (**b**) Situation before fat transplantation, lithotomy position, cranial view. (**c**) Situation after fat transplantation, overcorrection necessary

Pitfalls and Complications

When tightening or reduction of the labia majora is carried out in the same session as volume augmentation, the tissues are tightened first and the fat is not injected until after wound closure.

Although at first glance it may seem that reshaping the labia majora is less complicated than labia minora reduction, it is still not easy to achieve an aesthetically satisfactory result. The main reason is that the available options for remodelling the labia majora are restricted because of the lack of a firm fixation point and the ever-present risk of overcorrection with distortion and gaping of the introitus, as well as flattening and spreading of the inner labia. Volume replacement with autologous fat in some cases may require one or more repeat sessions before the desired effect is achieved.

Determining an indication for reduction of the labia majora should be more cautious than for the labia minora: weigh up the patient's expectations carefully against the realistic possibilities. On the other hand, volume augmentation with autologous fat grafting is a method that can be used readily, also in combination with labia minora reduction.

Labiaplasty of both the labia minora and the labia majora in one session is not advisable, as healing is made so much more difficult. Following combined procedures, the mechanical stresses from activities of daily living cause considerably more delayed wound healing and wound dehiscence and therefore affect the desired aesthetic outcome. The patient is often happy with a labia minora reduction alone, and no longer finds the original mild hyperplasia of the labia majora to be so bothersome. If reduction of both the inner and outer labia has to be carried out, the first step is to operate on the labia minora and not to perform the labia majora reduction until all the swelling has gone down, i.e. at least 6 months later.

Examples
Patient 1
Reductionplasty of the labia majora

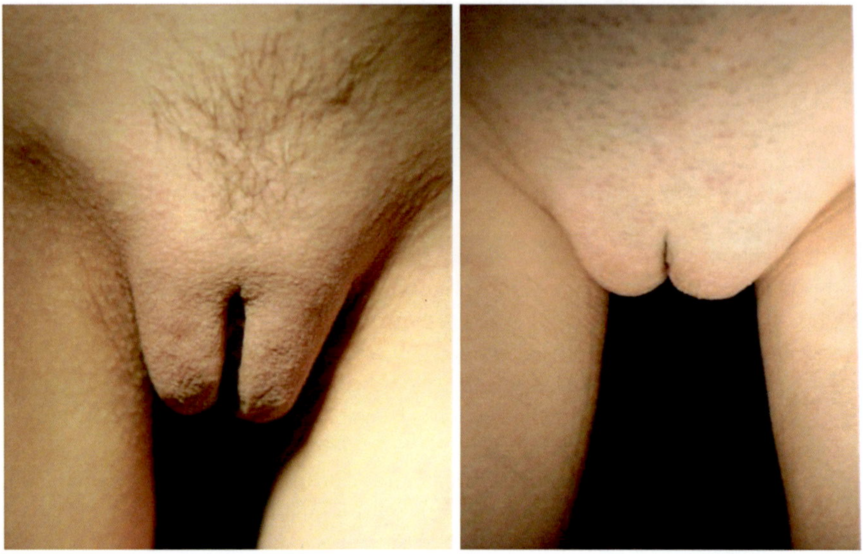

Patient 2
Reduction of the labia majora

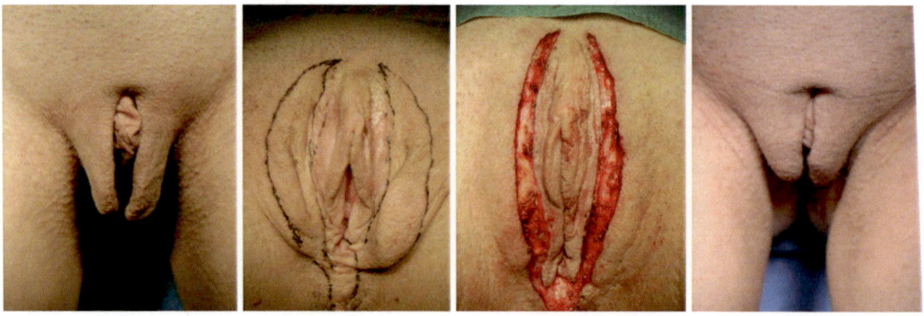

Patient 3
Reduction of the labia majora and minora

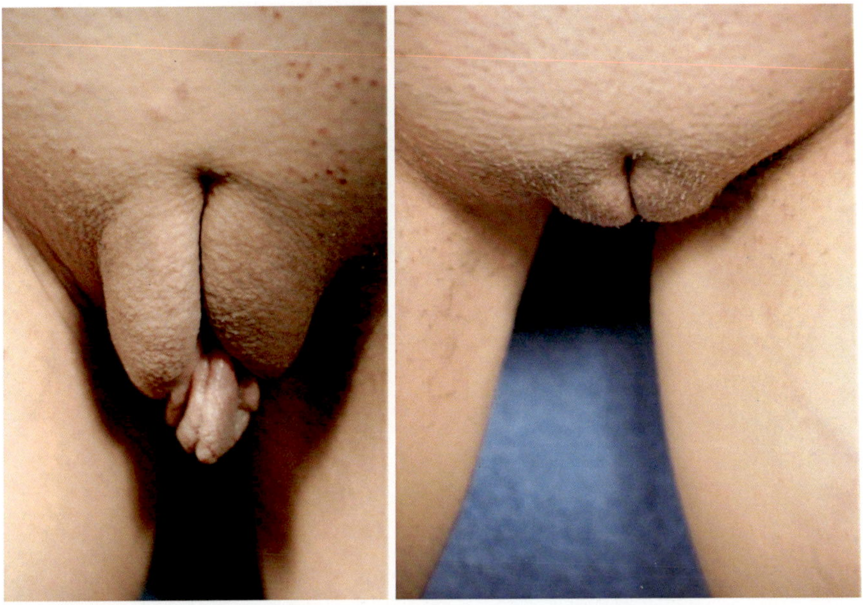

Patient 4
Reduction of labia majora and minora

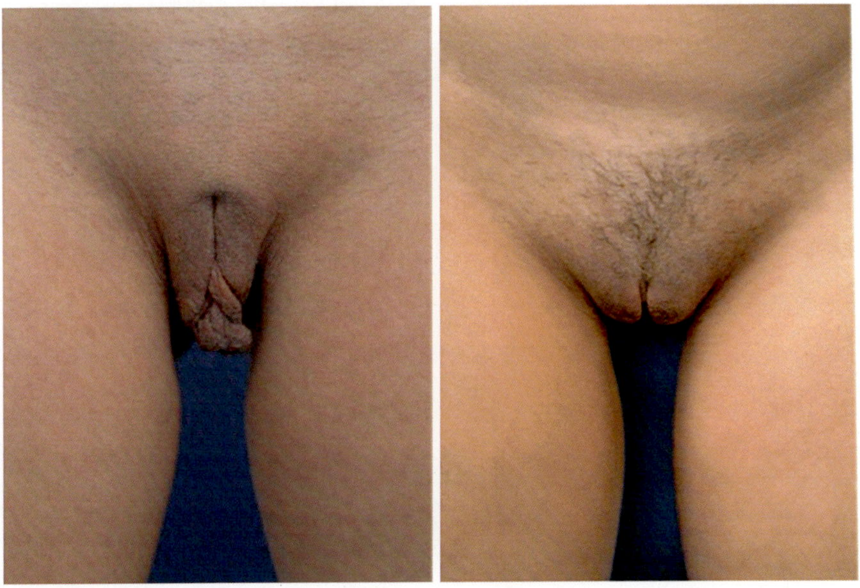

Patient 5
Reconstruction of the labia minora and lipostructure of labia majora

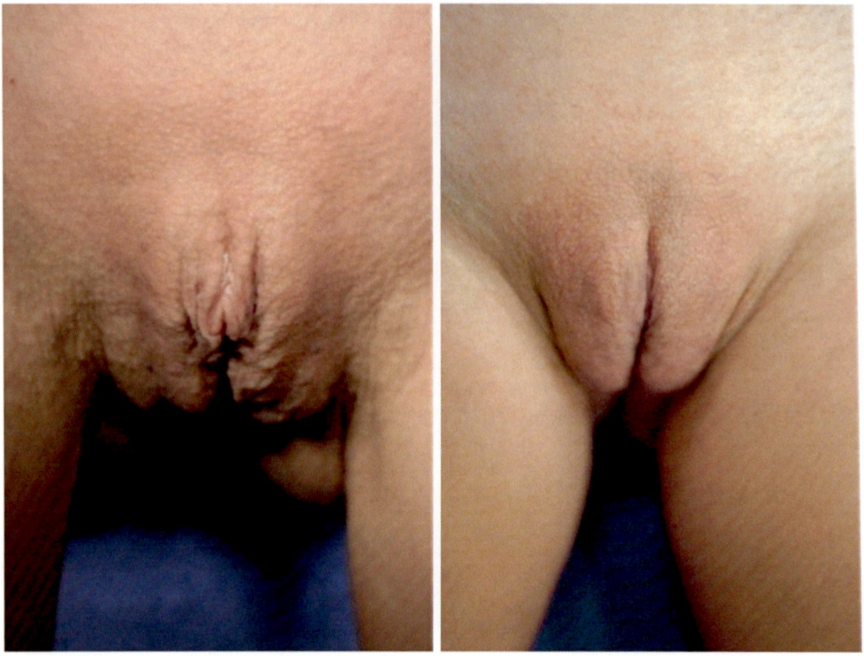

Patient 6
Reduction of the labia minora and lipostructure of the labia majora

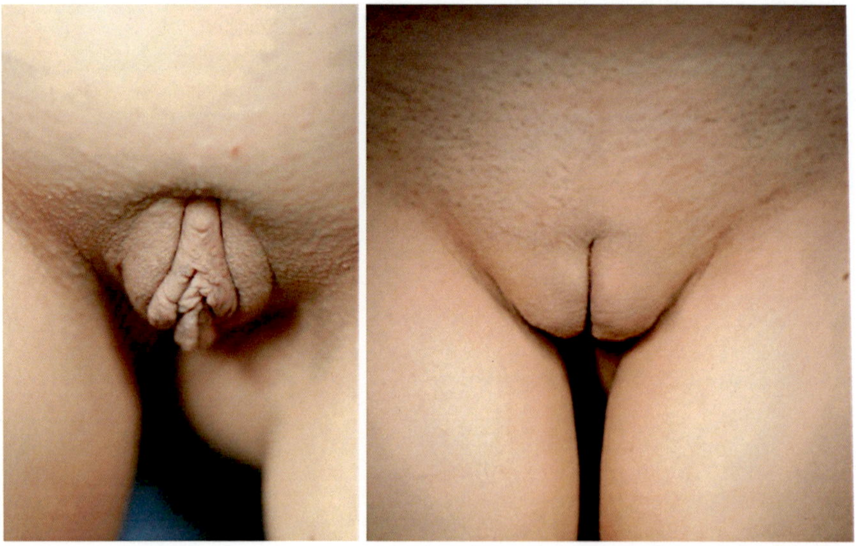

Mons Pubis

The superior border of the vulva is formed by the mons pubis. It is a gentle swelling beginning in the lower abdomen, extending downwards with a slight step to the origin of the labia majora. Laterally it flows almost seamlessly into the groin on both sides. Its curve and consistency is due to a cushion of fatty tissue beneath the relatively thick skin that is covered with pubic hair (Fig. 1).

Fat atrophy with age is usually less pronounced in the mons pubis than in the labia majora and may not even occur at all. On the contrary, the problem tends to be lipomatosis, often in combination with lax skin and descent of the mons pubis when it no longer sits firmly above the labia but slides forward over the superior origin of the labia majora.

There are rarely any functional problems, although, in some cases, pronounced changes may cause intertrigo: this is easy to treat with appropriate skin care and

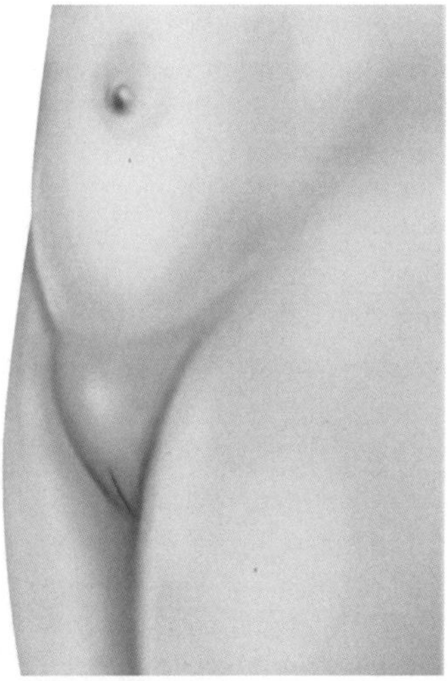

Fig. 1 Mons pubis

S. Gress, *Aesthetic and Functional Labiaplasty*,
DOI 10.1007/978-3-319-60222-6_5

clothing. The problem is usually visual. An adipose mons pubis bulges clearly when the patient is wearing a bikini or tight clothing.

Upwards tightening of the mons pubis and/or volume reduction by liposuction is the treatment of choice. In younger women, the skin is not usually so stretched and still has enough elasticity for liposuction alone to be adequate treatment for a moderate descent: the outcome is satisfactory without having to reckon with any troublesome excess skin after the procedure.

Liposuction

Every plastic surgeon is familiar with the technique of liposuction, so I need not go into detail here. Ultimately it makes no difference which method is preferred—classic tumescent technique or ultrasound liposuction—as long as it results in smooth regular contours. But that is not so easy over the relatively small surface area of the mons pubis.

Operation

The first step in the tumescent liposuction technique is to infiltrate the mons pubis with the tumescence solution, consisting of sodium chloride with added bicarbonate, lidocaine, and Suprarenin [adrenaline], via a small stab incision in the inguinal fold. This can be done with a pump or manually using a syringe. Close the incision with a suture so that the solution cannot flow out again, and allow about 15–20 min for the solution to be evenly distributed throughout the mons. With an adequate dose of lidocaine, the procedure can easily be carried out under local anaesthetic.

Suction out the fat through a stab incision about 3 mm long in the inguinal fold, working in a fan shape from each side, in order to achieve as smooth a result as possible without causing irregularities or dimples in the skin. For this reason, it is also important not to work too superficially but to leave a layer of fat about 0.5 cm thick under the skin (Fig. 2).

Close the incisions with a fine suture.

Postoperative Management

As after liposuction for any reason, an abdominal binder or firm control panties can be worn for a period of 4–6 weeks to provide compression in this region. The compression reinforces the even appearance of the skin and smooths out any minor irregularities in the contours. Skin care with a moisturising cream or lotion and gentle massage also help.

Any initial numbness of the skin over the mons pubis resolves within a few weeks.

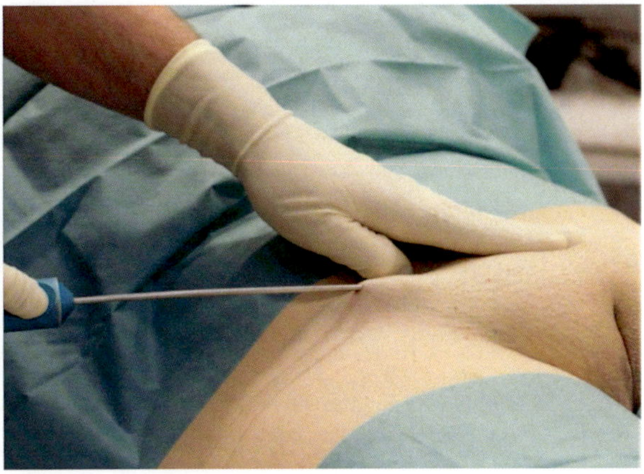

Fig. 2 Liposuction of the mons pubis via a lateral stab incision in the inguinal fold

Tightening Up the Mons Pubis

Shrinkage of the skin after liposuction is complete after about 6 months. Only then is it really possible to see if there is any residual excess skin. If, however, excess skin is to be expected after liposuction, tightening up of the mons pubis is indicated from the start.

Operation

The mons pubis is lifted by means of a spindle-shaped excision of the suprapubic skin, at about the level of a Pfannenstiel incision.

This procedure—also combined with liposuction—can easily be carried out under local anaesthetic. The width of the spindle determines the extent by which the skin is tightened. Depending on the findings, the spindle can be between 2 and 5 cm wide. To prevent distortion, make absolutely sure that the maximum width is right in the middle of the spindle and exactly in line with the pudendal cleft (Fig. 3a, b).

Close the wound with 3-0 absorbable sutures employing a continuous subcutaneous technique, leaving as few knots as possible to dissolve later. Subcutaneous knots may become obvious as reddened areas as they dissolve and later form scars.

Use 2-0 or 3-0 intradermal sutures to close the skin.

Postoperative Management

Adequate postoperative care consists of applying pressure to the scar and avoiding ultraviolet light for 6 months.

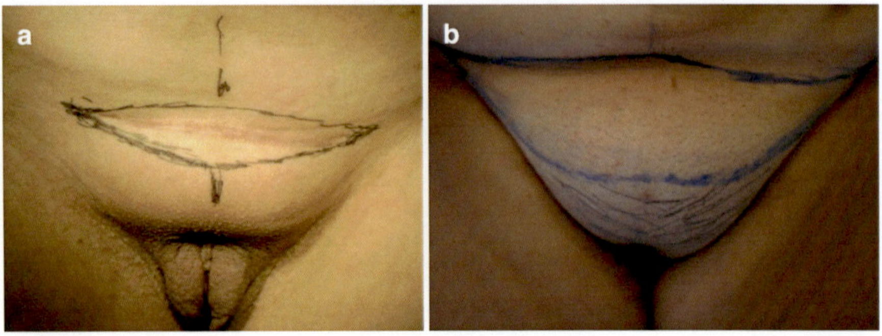

Fig. 3 (**a**) Marking the midline and the spindle to be excised; here with a c-section scar. (**b**) Large spindle for excision (*marked blue*), area for liposuction (*marked black*)

Examples
Patient 1
Liposuction and Lifting of the mons pubis, Liposuction of the abdomen

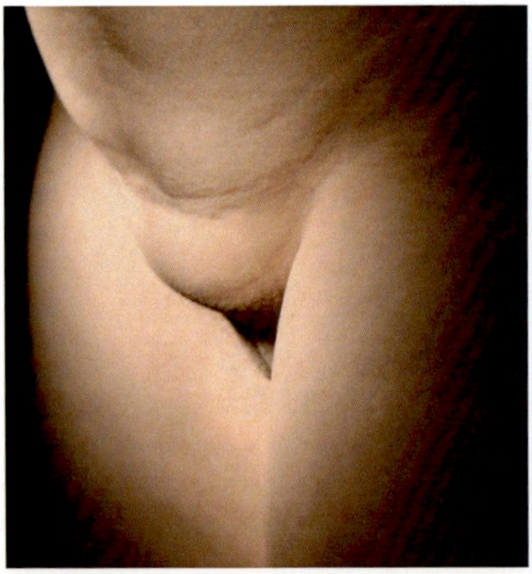

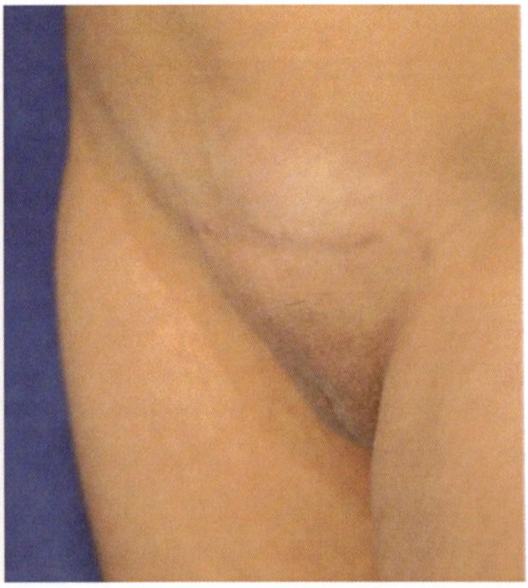

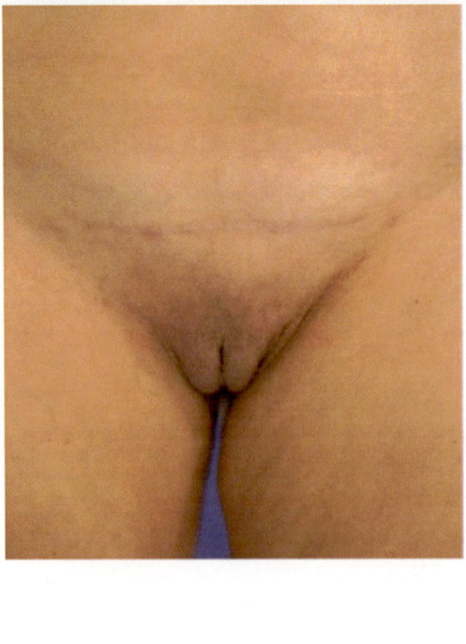

Patient 2

Liposuction and Lifting of the mons pubis. Abdominoplasty refused

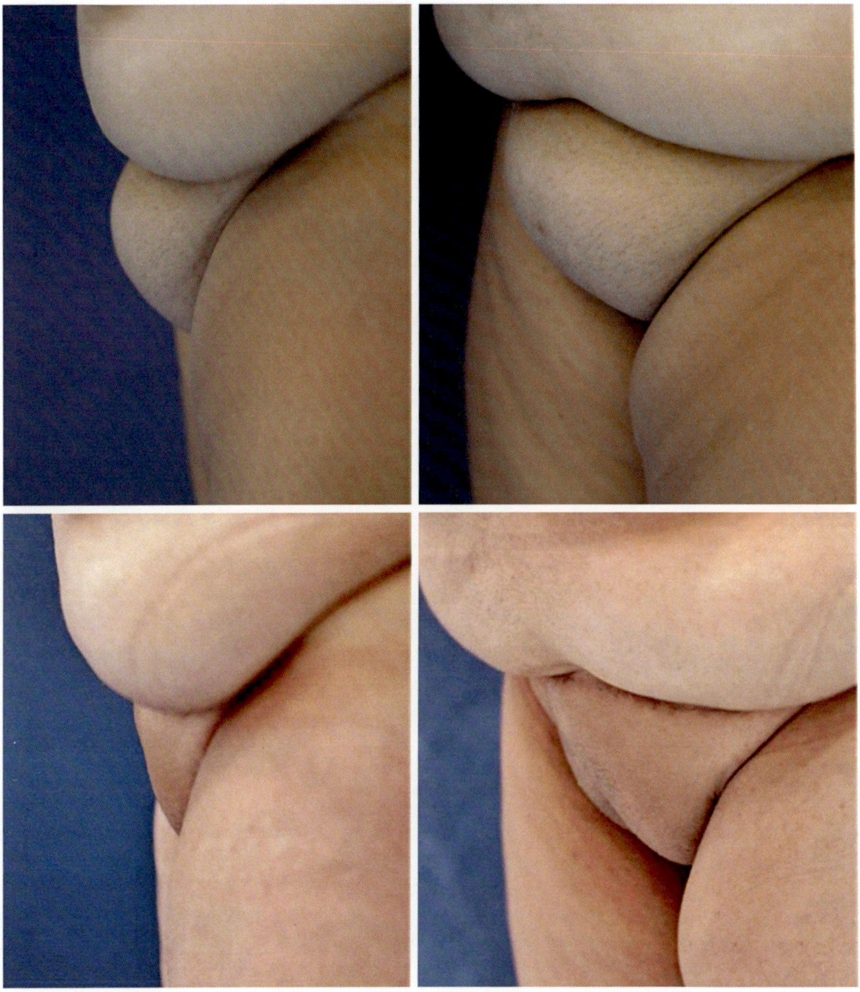

Patient 3
Liposuction of the mons pubis and abdomen

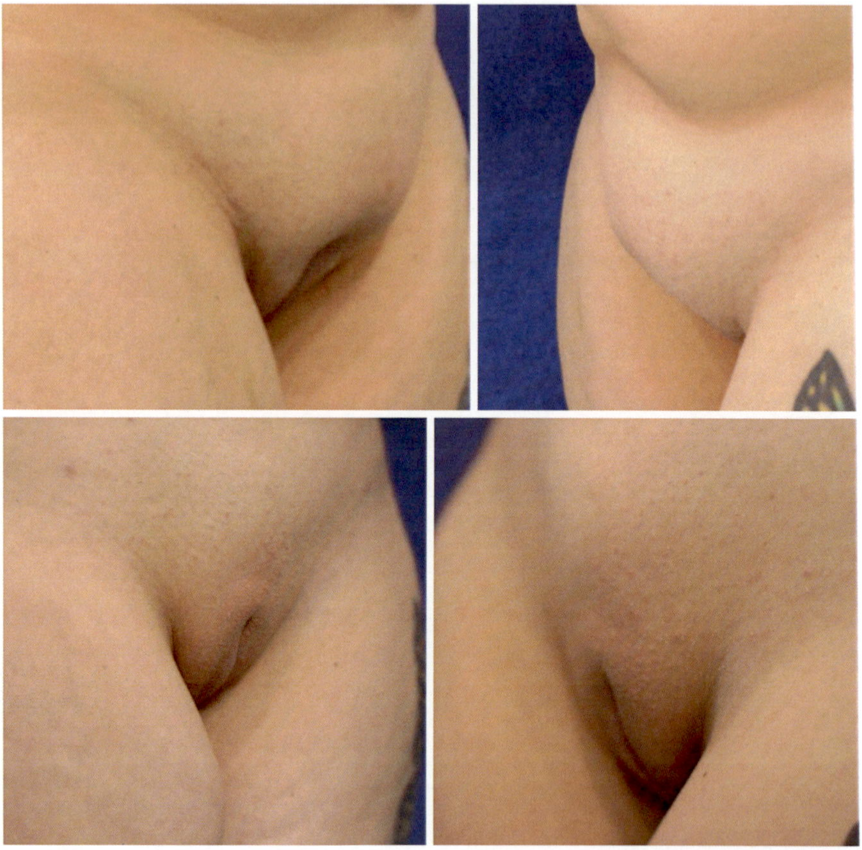

Afterword

In our short human existence, a great deal revolves around appreciation, especially when it comes to love and sexuality. They are the driving forces of many of our labours and the inspiration for music, poetry, and art. We therefore expend a good deal of our vital force and energy in striving for these ends.

When a person's lust for life diminishes, or disappears completely, an impairment or even complete loss of sexual drive is not infrequently responsible. There are numerous possible underlying reasons: advanced age, illness, marital or partnership problems, employment difficulties, etc. Another reason may be people's attitudes to themselves, especially with respect to their body image. How we perceive ourselves and our feelings has a great influence on our self-awareness and sexual identity, impacts on our sexual behaviour, and modifies the effects on possible partners.

The influences of body image on the soul and vice versa have been recognised since antiquity:

> "A change in the state of the soul alters the appearance of the body, and, conversely, when the appearance of the body changes, it alters the state of the soul as well."
>
> (Aristotle)

It is thus completely understandable that, on reaching the goal of all our efforts, we want to feel free and uninhibited to experience a fulfilling and satisfying sexuality in those moments reserved exclusively for that one special person. And part of it lies in our feeling content with our own physical appearance and our readiness to be seen naked. Surgical modifications of the genital area should do justice to these sensitive requirements, and surgeons who devote themselves to this field should be fully aware of them.

The term "intimate surgery", which is now being widely disseminated in the media, is a term indicating a path in medicine which perhaps includes new aspects and is not concerned only with serious illness; it is a path that addresses sexual questions, sensations, and the quality of intimate encounters. These are questions whose answers are not to be found in the realms of psychotherapy but rather require a surgical solution. But this doesn't only mean improvements in the appearance and functionality of the vulva, with all its individual components, as described in this book. It also means the function of vaginal sensation, restoring or even amplifying

S. Gress, *Aesthetic and Functional Labiaplasty*,
DOI 10.1007/978-3-319-60222-6

the response to sexual stimulation, especially after a woman has given birth or undergone any other lifetime change or disposition. And that should be the focus of development in female genital cosmetic surgery: there will be an increasing demand, and we should be ready to address it more closely.

My surgical colleagues who are active in this interesting field also have to meet the high requirements of their patients, in the same way as for any other procedures in plastic surgery. But they will also experience the gratitude and joy that come with targeted anatomical alterations that eliminate their patients' mental stress once and for all, and they can feel secure in the knowledge that they have helped their patients to realise a carefree and satisfying sexuality in the future.

Stefan Gress

Bibliography

Alter GJ (1998) New technique for aesthetic labia minora reduction. Ann Plast Surg 40:287–290

Alter GJ (2010) Labia minora reconstruction using clitoral hood flaps, wedge excisions, and YV advancement flaps. Plast Reconstr Surg 127(6):2356–2363

Baskin LS (2004) Anatomical studies of the female genitalia: surgical reconstructive implications. J Pediatr Endocrinol Metab 17:581–587

Baskin LS, Erol A, Wu LY, Kurzrock E, Cunha GR (1999) Anatomical studies of the human clitoris. J Urol 162:1025–1020

Bekker MD, Hogewoning C, Wallner C, Elzevier HW, DeRuiter MC (2012) The somatic and autonomic innervation of the clitoris; preliminary evidence of sexual dysfunction after minimally invasive slings. J Sex Med 9(6):1566–1578

Chavis WM, LaFerla JJ, Niccolini R (1989) Plastic repair of elongated, hypertrophic labia minors. A case report. J Reprod Med 34:373

Choi HY, Kim KT (2000) A new method for aesthetic reduction of labia minors (the deepithelialized reduction labiaplasty). Plast Reconstr Surg 105:419

Coleman SR (1995) Long-term survival of fat transplants: controlled demonstrations. Aesthetic Plast Surg 19:421

Coleman SR (2005) Structural fat grafting. Plast Reconstr Surg 115:1777

Cosson M (2004) Vaginale Chirurgie. Urban & Fischer, Munich, p 89

Di Marino V, Lepidi H (2014) Anatomic study of the clitoris and the bulbo-clitoral organ. Springer, Heidelberg

Dorschner W, Biesold M, Schmidt F, Stolzenburg JU (1999) The dispute about the external sphincter and the urogenital diaphragm. J Urol 162(6):1942–1945

Ellsworth WA, Rizvi M, Lypka M, Goan M, Smith B, Cohen B, Dinh T (2010) Techniques for labia minora reduction: an algorithmic approach. Aesthet Plast Surg 34:105–110Field LM (1991) Liposuction reduction of the suprapubic area. J Dermatol Surg Oncol 16:856

Foldes P, Buisson O (2009) The clitoral complex: a dynamic sonographic study. J Sex Med 6(5):1223–1231

Frick H, Leonhard H, Strack D (1980) Spezielle Anatomie II. Georg Thieme, München

Gilbert DA (1999) Female aesthetic genital surgery. In: Ehrlich RM, Alter GJ (eds) Reconstructive and plastic surgery of the external genitalia. WB Saunders, Philadelphia, p 471

Ginger VA, Cold CJ, Yang CC (2011) Surgical anatomy of the dorsal nerve of the clitoris. Neurourol Urodyn 30(3):412–416

Giraldo F, González C, De Haro F (2004) Central wedge nymphectomy with a 90-degree Z-plasty for aesthetic reduction of the labia minors. Plast Reconstr Surg 113:1820

Goldstein AMB, Padma-Nathan H (1990) The microarchitecture of the intracavernosal smooth muscle and the cavernosal fibrous skeleton. J Urol 144:1144–1146

Gravina GL, Brandetti F, Martini P et al (2008) Measurement of the thickness of the urethrovaginal space in women with or without vaginal orgasm. J Sex Med 5:610

Gray H (1978) Gray's anatomy of the human body, 29th edn. Lea & Febiger, Philadelphia, p 608

S. Gress, *Aesthetic and Functional Labiaplasty*,
DOI 10.1007/978-3-319-60222-6

Gress S (2007) Ästhetische und funktionelle Korrekturen im weiblichen Genitalbereich. Gynäkologisch-Geburtshilfliche Rundschau 47:23
Gress S (2013) Composite reduction labiaplasty. Aesthet Plast Surg 37:674–683
Hodgkinson DJ, Hait G (1984) Aesthetic vaginal labiaplasty. Plast Reconstr Surg 74:414
Honore LH, O'Hara KE (1978) Benign enlargement of the labia minora: report of two cases. Eur J Obster Gynecol Reprod Biol 8:61
Hruby S, Ebmer J, Dellon AL, Aszmann OC (2005) Anatomy of pudendal nerve at urogenital diaphragm—new critical site for nerve entrapment. Urology 66(5):949–952
Kantner M (1954) Studien über den sensiblen Apparat in der Glans clitoridis. (1. Die clitoris der Greisin). Ztschr Mikr Anat Forsch 60:388–398
Karacaoglu E (2005) The role of recipient sites in fat-graft survival. Ann Plast Surg 1:63
Köbelt GL (1851) De l´appariel du sens génital des deux sexes dans l´espèce humaine et dans quelques mammifères au point de vue anatomique et physiologique. Traduis de l´Allemand par Kaula H. Labé, Paris
Krizko M, Krizko M, Janek L (2005) Plastic adjustment in hypertrophy of labia minora (Slovak). Ceska Gynekol 70:446–449
Kruk-Jeromin J, Zielinski T (2010) Hypertrophy of labia minora: pathomorphology and surgical treatment. Ginekol Pol 81:298–302
Laub D (2000) A new method for aesthetic reduction of labia minors (the deepithelialized reduction labiaplasty) (discussion). Plast Reconstr Surg 105:423
Maas SM, Hage JJ (1998) Aesthetic labia minors reduction. Ann Plast Surg 41:685
Maas SM, Hage JJ (2000) Functional and aesthetic labia minors reduction. Plast Reconstr Surg 105:1453
Malionovsky L, Sommerova J, Martincik J (1975) Quantitative evaluation of sensory nerve endings in hypertrophy of labia minors pudenda in women. Acta Anatomica 92:129
Miklos JR, Moore RD (2003) Labiaplasty of the labia minora: patients´ indications for pursuing surgery. J Sex Med 5:1492–1495
Miklos JR, Moore RD (2012) Postoperative cosmetic expectations for patients considering labiaplasty surgery: our experience with 550 patients. Surg Technol Int 21:170–174
Mirilas P, Skandalakis JE (2004) Urogenital diaphragm: an erroneous concept casting its shadow over the sphincter urethrae and deep perineal space. J Am Coll Surg 198(2):279–290
Netter F (1987) Farbatlanten der Medizin 3 Genitalorgane. Georg Thieme, Stuttgart, p 90
Ngyen A, Pasky K (1990) Comparative study of survival of autologous adipose tissue taken and transplanted by different techniques. Plast Reconstr Surg 85:378
O'Connell HE, Eizenberg N, Rahman M, Cleeve J (2008) The anatomy of the distal vagina: towards unity. J Sex Med 5:1883–1891
O'Connell HE, Hutson J, Anderson CR, Plenter RJ (1998) Anatomical relationship between urethra and clitoris. J Urol 159(6):1892–1897
O'Connell HE, Hutson JM, Anderson CR, Plenter RJ, Hutson JM (2004) The clitoris: a unified structure. Histology of the clitoral glans, body, crura and bulbs. Urodinamica 14:127–132
O'Connell HE, Sanjeevan KV, Hutson JM (2005) Anatomy of the clitoris. J Urol 174(4 Pt 1 of 2):1189–1195
Oranges C, Sisti A, Sisti G (2015) Labia minora reduction techniques: a comprehensive literature review. Aesthet Surg J 35(4):419–431
Papagoeorgiou T, Hearns-Stokes R, Peppas D, Segars JH (2000) Clitorioplasty with preservation of neurovascular pedicles. Obstet Gynecol 96:821
Pernkopf E (1989) 2. Band, Topographische Anatomie des Menschen, Brust, Bauch und Extremitäten. Urban und Schwarzenberg, Wien-München
Platzer W (1985) Atlas of topographical anatomy. Georg Thieme, Stuttgart
Puppo V (2011) Review article anatomy of the clitoris: revision and clarifications about the anatomical terms for the clitoris proposed (without scientific bases) by Helen O'Connell, Emmanuele Jannini, and Odile Buisson
Radman HM (1976) Hypertrophy of the labia mionra. Obstet Gynecol 48(1 Suppl):78S–79S

Rees MA, O'Connell HE, Plenter RJ, Huston JM (2000) The suspensory ligament of the clitoris: connective tissue supports of the erectile tissues of the female urogenital region. Clin Anat 13:397–403

Rouzier R, Louis-Sylvestre C, Paniel BJ, Haddad B (2000) Hypertrophy of labia minora: experience with 163 reductions. Am J Obstet Gynecol 182:35–40

Sedy J, Nanka O, Spackova J, Jarolim L (2008) Clinical implications of a close vicinity of nervus dorsalis penis/clitoridis and os pubis. J Sex Med 5(7):1572–1581

Shaw A (1977) Subcutaneous reduction clitoroplasty. J Pediatr Surg 12:331

Sobotta J (1982) Atlas der Anatomie des Menschen 2. Urban & Schwarzenberg, München

Solanski NS, Trejero-Trujeque R, Stevens-King A, Matala CM (2010) Aesthetic and functional reduction of the labia minora using the Maas and Haage technique. J Plast Reconstr Aesthet Surg 63:1181–1185

Stein TA, DeLancey JOL (2008) Structure of perineal membrane in females: gross and microscopic anatomy. Obstet Gynecol 111(3):686–693

Suh DD, Yang CC, Cao Y, Garland PA, Maravilla KR (2003) Magnetic resonance imaging anatomy of the female genitalia in premenopausal and postmenopausal women. J Urol 170:138–144

Trichot C, Thubert T, Faivre E, Fernandez H, Deffieux X (2011) Surgical reduction of hypertrophy of the labia minora. Int J Gynaecol Obsts 115(1):40–43

Vaze A, Goldman H, Jones JS, Rackley R, Vasavada S, Gustavson KJ (2009) Determining the course of the dorsal nerve of the clitoris. Urology 72(5):1040–1043

Winkelmann RK (1959) The erogenous zones: their nerve supply and significance. Mayo Clin Proc 34(2):39–47

Yilmaz U, Kromm BG, Yang CC (2004) Evaluation of autonomic innervation of the clitoris and bulb. J Urol 172(5 Pt 1):1930–1934. discussion 1934

Yj C, Li FY, Zhou CD, Hu JT, Ding J, Xie LH, Li SK (2012) A modified method of labia minora reduction: the deepithelialised reduction of the central and posterior labia minora. J Plast Reconstr Aesthet Surg 65(8):1096–1102

Yucel S, De Souza A Jr, Baskin LS (2004) Neuroanatomy of the human female lower urogenital tract. J Urol 172(1):191–195

Zeitfracht Medien GmbH
Ferdinand-Jühlke-Straße 7
99095 Erfurt, Deutschland
produktsicherheit@kolibri360.de